The Diploma in Child Health

A practical study guide
Volume 1

By Dr Anil Garg, Dr Siba Prosad Paul,
Dr Geethika Bandaranayake,
Dr Urmilla Pillai and Dr Neelu Garg

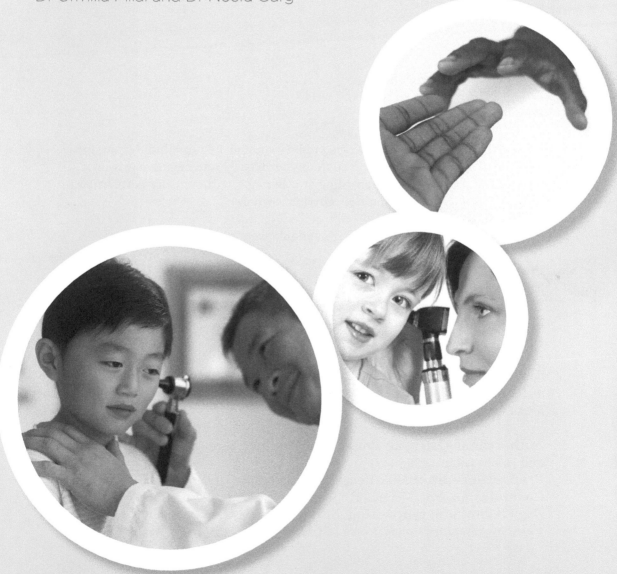

Diploma in Child Health: A practical study guide, volume 1

Published by:
Pavilion Publishing and Media Ltd
Rayford House
School Road
Hove
East Sussex
BN3 5HX
Tel: 01273 434 943
Fax: 01273 227 308
Email: info@pavpub.com

Published 2014

A catalogue record for this book is available from the British Library.

Print ISBN: 978-1-909810-60-0
Epub ISBN: 978-1-909810-61-7
PDF ebook ISBN: 978-1-909810-62-4
Kindle ISBN: 978-1-909810-63-1

Pavilion is the leading training and development provider and publisher in the health, social care and allied fields, providing a range of innovative training solutions underpinned by sound research and professional values. We aim to put our customers first, through excellent customer service and value.

Authors: Anil Garg, Siba Prosad Paul, Geethika Bandaranayake, Urmila Pillai and Neelu Garg
Production editor: Mike Benge, Pavilion Publishing and Media Ltd
Cover design: Phil Morash, Pavilion Publishing and Media Ltd
Page layout and typesetting: Emma Dawe, Pavilion Publishing and Media Ltd
Printing: Ashford Colour Press Ltd, Gosport, Hampshire

Contents

Focused history and management station

Child development station

Preface

The DCH examination consists of both written and clinical components, and this book and its counterpart, Volume 2, are intended to help candidates prepare for the clinical examination and guide you through the various stations you will encounter.

I would suggest you use the guides to practise under examination conditions and not use them as bedtime reading. The cases are real and cover a wide cross-section of potential topics. It is important to note that the books are not intended to be textbooks, and although they supply some basic information on the topics covered, you will need to do some extensive supportive reading.

This is Volume 1, which covers the stations common to both the DCH and the MRCPCH examinations. Volume 2 covers the remaining stations that will be covered in the DCH exam.

I hope you find the books helpful to your preparations for the examination, and stimulating and informative reads.

I would like to take this opportunity to thank all of my colleagues who have contributed to these books and acknowledge the hard work they have put in to make them possible.

Remember, there is always room for improvement – practise, practise, practise…

Dr Anil Garg

Foreword

It is a pleasure to write a foreword to this book, which I'm sure will be warmly welcomed by junior doctors preparing for the DCH clinical examination. This examination is important for doctors wanting to demonstrate competency in looking after children in primary care settings, and for that reason is a valuable qualification to obtain.

The most recent format of the examination came into force in 2011, introducing new stations including safe prescribing, data interpretation and structured oral stations. The examination circuit is completed by having assessments of clinical skills, neurodisability and development and communication.

I found it interesting that the authors have decided to publish this book in two volumes, separating out the stations unique to the DCH clinical examination in one volume and having the stations common to that and the MRCPCH clinical examination in the other.

Together, these books provide a valuable resource for anyone preparing for the DCH examination, and Volume 1 will be a helpful tool for those taking the MRCPCH exam, as each station is considered separately and many clinical scenarios are presented within each section.

Anna Mathew
Consultant Paediatrician
Western Sussex hospitals NHS Trust, UK

Introduction: The DCH examination

Children are a vulnerable part of society. They differ from adults in a number of ways, starting out as helpless and totally dependent on their carers for survival, and they have different needs due to the demands of growth and development. Although, comparatively, they make up a smaller proportion of the population than adults, they require much higher levels of care. Their needs are often quite specific and the people caring for them need special skills to provide for them.

The Diploma in Child Health (DCH) is a qualification that recognises that the holder has achieved the competencies and skills required to look after children. The examination has evolved over the years, both in format and in relevance. In the UK, it used to be the only qualification in paediatrics for hospital specialists taken after getting the Membership of the College of Physicians (MRCP). However, with the inception by Royal Charter in 1996 of the RCPCH (Royal College of Paediatrics and Child Health), membership of RCPCH (ie. the MRCPCH exams) established a second specialist qualification in addition to the DCH that confirms and attests a speciality in paediatrics.

The DCH used to be an examination run by hospital paediatricians for hospital paediatricians. In the UK, however, it has evolved into an examination oriented towards primary care and general practice. According to the RCPCH, the DCH is now designed to recognise competence in the care of children in general practitioner vocational trainees, staff grade doctors and senior house officers in paediatrics, as well as trainees in specialties allied to paediatrics.

The examination has a syllabus that encompasses paediatric care both in and out of hospital, plus services available and used outside the hospital settings. Examiners include hospital paediatricians, community paediatricians, general practitioners, paediatric surgeons and child psychiatrists.

This change in emphasis is important. In terms of the workload in primary care for a GP, children contribute approximately 30%, significantly more than their number in the community. GPs need to work with numerous agencies now involved in the multidisciplinary approach to childcare, and they need to recognise when to seek assistance from the appropriate agencies.

A busy GP has to manage children with acute and chronic conditions, monitor their development, discuss health promotion and be aware of child protection issues and various other screening programmes. They also have to be aware of the resources available and how to tap them for the benefit of children they are looking after. Competence and confidence in dealing with them and their conditions is therefore vital.

The Diploma in Child Health is an accepted specialist qualification overseas. Hence it is important to have adequate experience of hospital paediatrics to pass the examination in the various domains: clinical, communication, history and management, development, prescribing and structured oral.

The safe prescribing station is a new domain in the exam, and has been introduced to improve prescribing skills and prevent harm to patients. Prescribing errors are in fact a leading cause of death in young adults between 18–45 years, after accidents. And it is not only prescribing errors, but errors in dispensing due to illegibility that also contribute to the total damage, hence the need for improvement. When prescribing, it is important to use the British National Formulary for Children (BNFC) to check for appropriate drug choice, dosage, side effects and interactions. There may be local guidelines available that can be used instead.

Candidates taking the DCH examination overseas must be aware of the management and support provided to children in the community in which they practise. They should read up and be aware of the management and support that is available in the UK. This will often not be available overseas, but it can be quoted as best practice and what should be aspired to in the future, and contrasted with what is actually available.

The structure of the exam

The DCH examination consists of two parts:

Foundation of Practice: Part 1. This is the written component and is the same as that for MRCPCH. There are two papers consisting of multiple choice, extended matching and best-of-five format questions. The written questions are prepared and checked in different settings before being used in the examination. After each diet, the performance of each question is evaluated and each question is given a score. Poorly discriminating questions are not used in the future.

Clinical examination: Part 2. This is the practical component of the examination and has been included since 2006. It has evolved from a format that included a long case, short cases and viva, to an OSCE (Objective Structured Clinical Examination) format, which is more consistent in assessment, fairer to candidates and has improved accountability. A number of candidates are assessed in the same 'station/skill set' by the same examiner with the same patient, to provide better consistency in assessment and grading.

The RCPCH puts a great deal of effort into ensuring that every examination is of a comparable standard to the last and is thorough and fair. Setting standards is an important part of ensuring fairness and equality across the various centres hosting the examination. It involves deciding on what is expected of the candidate with reference to the anchor statements as published by the RCPCH. The communication and prescribing scenarios are 'standard set' at the RCPCH, and guidance is given to the centres hosting the examination, thus reducing variability in assessment.

Before an exam, the examiners are given a written summary of the signs and symptoms of the clinical cases who are to be investigated during the examination. Children are then assessed at the examination centre for the validity of these symptoms and a standard is set by two examiners, who determine what is expected of a candidate in order to achieve a particular grade from 'clear pass' to 'clear fail'. 'Unacceptable' is reserved for rare cases. These standard setting forms are returned to the RCPCH at the end of the examination.

The stations

In the DCH clinical examination, skills and competence are assessed in seven different areas at eight stations. These cover:

- communication
- focused history and management
- structured oral
- clinical assessment
- child development
- data interpretation
- safe prescribing.

The eight OSCE stations are divided into two circuits – separated as follows:

Circuit A (lasts 36 minutes): each station lasts six minutes with a three-minute interval between stations.

Circuit B (lasts 48 minutes): each station lasts nine minutes with a three-minute interval between stations.

The candidates move from station to station while the examiner remains at the same station during the session. This provides consistency in examining and marking the performance of the candidates against the standard that was set before the start of the session.

There is a 40 minute break between the two circuits.

12 objective assessments are made of each candidate. One assessment is made at each station in Circuit A (for a total of four assessments), and two assessments are made at each station in Circuit B (for a total of eight assessments).

Circuit A grid

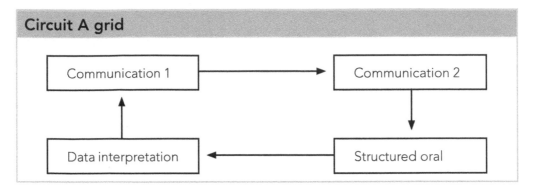

Time frame for Circuit A

Station	Interval outside	In station	Warning
Communication 1	Scenario available Read and make plan	6 minute assessment	1 minute remaining
Communication 2	Scenario available Read and make plan	6 minute assessment	1 minute remaining
Data interpretation	No information available outside	2 minutes to interpret data 4 minute discussion with examiner	1 minute remaining
Structured oral	No information available outside	1–2 minutes to read scenario 4–5 minutes discussion with examiner	1 minute remaining

For more information, visit www.rcpch.ac.uk/examinations/dch

Circuit B grid

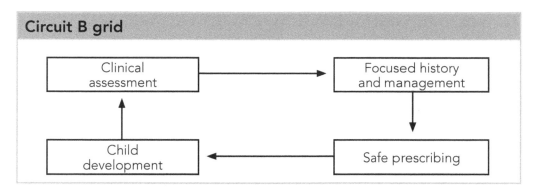

Time frame for Circuit B

Station	Interval outside	In station	Warning
Clinical assessment	None	Assessment of child 6 min Discussion with examiner 3 min	1 minute remaining
Focused history/ management	Scenario to read *Read and make plan*	6 min with role player Role player leaves 3 min discuss with examiner	4 minutes remaining
Development	None	6 min assess child 3 min discuss with examiner	4 minutes remaining
Prescribing	Task description *Read and make plan*	5 minute to write prescription 4 min discussion with examiner	5 minutes remaining

Note – Two sets of marks are awarded for each station (for task and discussion)

Marking schedule

Grade	Marks	Description
Clear Pass (CP)	12	Satisfied requirements and excelled
Pass	10	Some minor failings – not as good as expected
Bare fail	8	Inappropriate number of minor or some important errors
Clear fail	4	Poor performance
Unacceptable	0	Unprofessional behaviour – rough, rude

Total of 120 marks are needed in examination to be awarded a pass.

Clinical examination station

The following are some examples of tasks that you might be asked to perform at the clinical examination station:

A: 'Please examine Peter's chest. He is eight years old and has come for review due to his recurrent cough.'

B: 'Please examine Anu, five years old, who had a murmur noted during a febrile illness four weeks ago.'

C: 'Joanna is seven years old and her mother is worried about her walking, believing she has a limp. Please examine Joanna's legs.'

D: 'Daniel, six years old, has come for review as his mother feels he is not as good with his hands as his twin sister. Can you please do a fine motor assessment?'

The examiner will complete the mark sheet as the candidate proceeds with the task at the station, and will write comments about the performance for later feedback and in case there are any questions as to why a certain mark was given.

Data interpretation station

Data interpretation is a new station in the DCH, which tests the ability of a candidate to assess the results of investigations in a clinical setting. The data interpretation station has one scenario only, which will consist of a set of results from a haematology or biochemistry report, for example, or from an audiogram or a renogram etc. The candidate's task is to interpret the data provided, work out a differential diagnosis if appropriate, devise a management plan and discuss it with the examiner.

It is rare for identical questions to appear but there are recurring themes.

Marks are awarded against a pre-determined standard, and will assess whether a candidate:

■ identifies the problem

■ accurately interprets the data in the clinical context provided

■ achieves the correct diagnosis or a differential diagnosis

■ is fluent and confident in discussing management of the condition

■ demonstrates their knowledge underpinning good paediatric practice

■ demonstrates a good understanding of the evidence base ie. NICE guidelines.

There is no substitute for a broad knowledge base and an ability to think laterally. Remember, the data could either be normal or could indicate significant pathology.

Safe prescribing station

Safe prescribing is a station for assessing the understanding of pharmacological agents, other compounds, devices and measures used in managing disease conditions, both acute and chronic. A clinical scenario is given and the candidate has to prescribe the most appropriate drug or device. Competences assessed include the correct use of medication/intervention in the right medical context and in the correct dosage. The candidate has to decide on the most appropriate strategy and write out a prescription with the help of the BNFC (British National Formulary for Children) (if overseas, local guidelines may be used). This is followed by a discussion with the examiner.

Latest updates can be obtained from the RCPCH – http://www.rcpch.ac.uk/Examinations/DCH

The structure of this study manual

In the subsequent sections of this study manual we will cover the following stations:

- Communication

- Clinical assessment

- Focused history and management

- Child development

In *The Diploma in Child Health: A practical study guide, Volume 2*, the remaining stations are covered. These are:

- Safe prescribing

- Data interpretation

- Structured oral

The books have been divided in this way because the stations covered in this manual are common to both the DCH exam and the MRCPCH exam, and this book is therefore of relevance to candidates taking either. The stations covered by Volume 2 are only relevant to the DCH.

The difference between the DCH and MRCPCH examinations lies in the degree of competence expected, which is reflected in the time allocated for testing competencies at each station.

The scenario-based approach that is used in this manual keeps in perspective that the candidate is a new GP in the UK who has four to six months' of working in paediatrics and other specialities during their two years' hospital-based training and one year in general practice. During this time, the individual will have acquired other common and transferrable competences from the various other specialities they have developed through their vocational training.

The scenarios in this manual are generally designed to be practised with another person who can act as a 'role player', either playing the part of the patient or their parent, or the examiner in scenarios where you will have to discuss your findings. The information for each scenario is therefore divided into different sections, some of which both you and your partner will have access to, and the rest which will only be available to the role player.

In scenarios where the role player is playing the examiner, they will essentially have the 'answers', and a list of areas that the examiner will be looking for.

The scenarios are presented in four sections, each in a different coloured box:

- The first box sets the scene and outlines the task you need to perform as the candidate.

- The information in the second box will vary depending on the station. It will contain either:

    - the information given to the role player, which should not be available to the candidate

    - further, more detailed information for the candidate, such as a set of data to be interpreted or the details of a clinical examination.

- The third box, which should not be available to the candidate, contains information about what the examiner expects of a candidate and, usually, the 'answers' or conclusions that the candidate would be expected to reach.

- The fourth box contains some further basic information on the topic that may be useful for other stations, or that might simply further the candidates understanding of the topic.

- Finally, there is a small space for you to make notes that come to mind.

We therefore recommend that you do not use the book as a passive reading material, but work through it with friends in small study groups using the book as a guide.

However, if you do not have a study partner you can still work through the scenarios by simply covering up or ignoring those boxes that contain information for the role player, and writing down your responses, diagnoses and thoughts. These can then be checked against the information or answers in the remaining boxes.

Further video resources to help you can be found at www.mrcpchclinicals.org

General approach to the examination

By their very nature, examinations are very artificial situations, far removed from the day-to-day routines we all are so accustomed to. On a normal day, one would come to work and get on with the tasks as they arise: handover, ward round, admitting, taking a history from a parent or patient and working out a management plan, multidisciplinary meeting, talking to children or parents, and if there is more than one job to be done, we prioritise. Sometimes we might demonstrate our skills to our junior colleagues for them to learn, or to seniors to get their feedback with a view to improving and providing better care to our patients, but generally we are not concerned about who is watching us and we do not have to show our best side.

Examinations, however, are different. Think of the driving test you may have taken. It was not only about your driving; you had to 'exaggerate' your actions – adjusting the rear view mirror before starting, constantly checking mirrors and making sure it was noted by the examiner. It was not simply what you were doing that mattered, but also about *showing*, and ensuring that what you had been doing was noted.

Clinical examinations in general, and the DCH in particular, are not miles away from this. You have to 'perform', and to show off your various skills and competences in the different settings of the examination stations, be it communication with parents or a child or both, discussing with a colleague, taking a focused history, interpreting a result, or writing a prescription.

I, like most people, feel uncomfortable when I am being observed critically while doing something. It makes me nervous and jittery. In a work environment I can request an observer – such as a parent whose child is undergoing a lumbar puncture or a venepuncture – to kindly leave and wait outside while I complete the task. One does not have that option during an examination. Being observed is part of the deal we have agreed to, and coping with the nerves is an important factor in the final outcome.

Your preparation for the DCH examination will culminate at the examination centre, but should start much earlier: check out the route to the centre the night before, get a good night's sleep, leave yourself plenty of time to get ready, dress in a conservative style and present a professional image. Stay calm on the way to the examination centre and get there in good time as any delay or potential delays will increase your tension and anxiety, adversely affecting your ability to perform at your best.

As discussed, there are eight stations to negotiate during the examination and it is very unlikely that all of them will go completely to your satisfaction. There will be times when you think you have 'bombed' a particular station and the feeling is devastating. But it is very important not to lose your cool and go to pieces. My boss used to say, take it like a game of cricket – each station is one wicket – just because one or even two wickets fall with not enough score on the board, it does not mean the game is lost. Keep your head down, keep your concentration and try and score in the next station/wicket. The previous station cannot affect the next if you do not let it, and marks from one station can compensate for the other stations and take you to the desired total to pass. You should therefore never give up!

Communication is key to this examination. It is important in all sections and stations. You will be replying to questions throughout the examination. It is important to have a strategy that will guide you through most situations and keep you in control.

'That is a very good question!' is probably not the best response to come out with in the examination, though you may hear it time and again in the media.

Here are some essential tips.

■ Do not be tempted to speak immediately after the question has been asked.

■ Do not say the first thing that comes to mind – other ideas may not follow.

■ Take up to 10 seconds to think over a question carefully.

■ Work out precisely what is being asked.

■ Differentiate from what you think you would like to have heard.

■ Think of three common points in relation to the question asked.

■ If possible, think of the next question that may follow on from your answer.

■ Try to guide the examiner to areas you know well.

■ If it so happens that you do not know enough about a particular condition, do not mention it – as long as it is not the first on the list.

■ If pressed, admit your lack of knowledge and the examiner will move on – do not bluff – examiners are seasoned players.

■ When you do start replying, keep your thoughts five seconds ahead of your mouth. With practice this is possible, difficult as it may seem now. Practising the scenarios in this manual with friends/study partners will get you used to this.

■ Finally, if you are not sure of what is being asked – CLARIFY.

You may think that an initial five to 10-second silence is long, awkward and feels like eternity, but trust me, a 10-second silence in the middle of a sentence, when the ideas you want to convey are at the tip of your tongue but just won't come, is a lot more awkward and 'deafening'. You can try it with a recording.

This emphasis on communication is not 'overkill', and the time you spend now on practising and improving this skill will help you more than anything else you may do so close to the exam.

Remember, practice makes perfect – failing to prepare is preparing to fail.

We hope you find the book useful and interesting.

Communication station

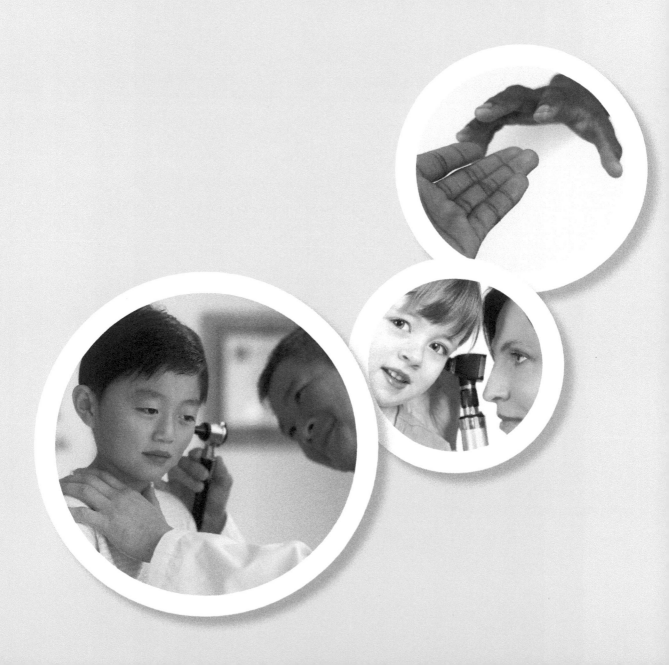

Communication station

Communication in the DCH

There are two stations in the DCH examination that focus on communication, signifying the importance that the RCPCH attributes to this skill in a doctor. These stations are set up to replicate the interaction between a doctor and a patient, or a doctor and a medical colleague or other team member, such as a nurse, student or manager.

This interaction could be in an outpatient clinic, it could be a consultation, a review on or following a ward round, a demonstration of a medical device or a meeting with a parent to address their concerns.

Relational versatility is the ability of a physician/doctor to match their interpersonal approach to different patient's needs; to be able to be who and what a patient needs as the need arises, such as when a 'routine' appointment turns out to require the delivery of bad news with life changing implications. It is built upon an attitude of mutual respect and treating others how we would like to be treated ourselves. It involves the capacity to observe ourselves as others, to see and 'experience' an interaction with us.

The majority of tasks in the doctor–patient relationship are carried out by verbal communication. A patient comes with their problems expecting a solution, or hoping for their concerns to be addressed. During a consultation, doctor and patient commonly rely on a shared language to explore concerns, build a timeline history and to interpret cues. Communication styles need to be adapted to an individual patient's needs as the consultation progresses, so as to fully understand the patient's concerns, and then discuss the various management options. This should really be a two-way process, but was observed by Roter and Larson (2002) to be 'largely a physician monologue', but it ignored the experiences of the doctor and to an extent the emotional context of the interaction.

There are other dimensions also in play during any medical encounter or consultation.

- How the participants (doctor and patient) feel about each other.
- Who assumes and leads.
- The emotional agreement on the treatment.

It is important to remember, however, that communication is less verbal and more about the associated softer qualities of an interaction.

Nonverbal communication is integral and vital to interactions between patient and doctor, and includes our bodies: face-to-face exchanges, facial expressions, posture and dress, all of which can modify and support what we say verbally, or can even contradict our verbal message. Eye contact, for example, can reflect a variety of things including attentiveness, a challenge to authority or a lack of interest.

The tone of what we say can be accurately recognised with remarkable accuracy by patients, who can predict outcomes on the basis of voice tones alone during simulated sessions.

Although some of our attitudes and behaviours are deliberate and can be consciously employed, much is a spontaneous expression of our attitudes, values and inner feelings, and we cannot effectively put on a 'show'.

The art of medicine lies in its 'soft' side, which doctors are taught to develop during their training and subsequent career to improve the care they provide. Being so fundamental to the practice of medicine, it is also rigorously tested in the DCH at the communication and history and management stations, and plays a significant part in the clinical assessment, safe prescribing, structured oral and data interpretation stations, when we communicate with the examiner.

Makoul (2001) provides a very clear framework to guide a consultation that is clearly signposted, and the elements of this framework are also used in the DCH assessment.

These elements divide a medical consultation into the following seven domains.

- The doctor–patient relationship – building rapport – fundamental task

- Opening the discussion

- Gathering information

- Understanding the patient's perspective

- Sharing information

- Agreeing problems and plans

- Providing closure

Building a rapport:

The first task here is fundamental, and all subsequent actions depend on the ability to build a relationship and rapport with the patient in an atmosphere of mutual trust where information, often of a sensitive nature, may be divulged.

The most important thing for obtaining a positive relationship with the patient is to listen attentively and provide reassurance. This remains the case throughout the consultation process.

Opening the discussion:

■ Allow the patient to complete their opening statement – do not interrupt.

■ Elicit a full set of concerns.

■ Establish and maintain a personal connection.

Gathering information:

■ Use open-ended and closed questions appropriately.

    ■ How are you feeling today?

    ■ What did you do at school today?

    ■ How do you make your breathing better?

    ■ How can I help?

    ■ Do you have fever?

    ■ Do you take your medicine regularly?

    ■ Did you take your medicine today?

■ Structure, clarify and summarise information.

    ■ Ask for information to be repeated.

    ■ Summarise yourself and check there is concurrence.

■ Actively listen using nonverbal and verbal cues.

    ■ Eye contact.

    ■ Nod.

    ■ Words of encouragement – 'Umm', 'Yes', 'I see'.

Understanding the patient's perspective

■ A worried patient will need information in a reassuring and supportive manner.

■ Patients with low self-esteem need praise, respect, support and guidance to resources.

■ If a patient is asking for superfluous investigations (an MRI scan, for example) or treatments, establish their motives and thoroughly understand their wishes before making any decision.

- Angry patients require acceptance and containing functions.
- Explore contextual factors, such as:
  - family
  - culture
  - socioeconomic status.
- Explore beliefs, concerns and expectations about health and illness.
  - 'How would you like to feel?'
  - 'What's worrying you about your illness?'
- Acknowledge and respond to the patient's ideas, feelings and values:
  - 'I see this is obviously troubling you a great deal – perhaps we can do...'
  - 'You are concerned about your son's school attendance – why?'

Sharing information:

- Use language the patient can understand – start with the level of a 10-year-old.
- Check understanding:
  - build up or down depending on response
  - put information in the context of a patient's sphere of knowledge.

Agreeing problems and plans:

- Encourage the patient to participate in decisions as they are more likely to comply.
- Check the patient's willingness to follow a plan.
- Check the patient's ability to follow a plan.
- Identify and list any resources and support available:
  - possible out-reach services
  - support groups
  - leaflets.

Providing closure:

- Ask if the patient has any other issues or concerns.
- Summarise and affirm agreement with the plan of action.
- Explain plans to children in age-appropriate language.

Diploma in Child Health: Volume 1 © Pavilion Publishing and Media Ltd and its licensors 2014.

ediatric three-way consultation

patients are children, but it will primarily be their parents who will be anxious, ried, and who will ask most of the questions. We therefore have to develop skills to be able to engage **both** child and parent appropriately. It is always ꞁortant to interact with the child and include them in the discussion as much as ꞁible. **Ignore the child at your peril**. If a child is present, start by interacting ꞁ them using an opening, welcoming remark or introducing yourself and asking estion they should be able to answer, such as 'What did you do at school ꞁerday?' or 'What do you like best at school?' You can then move on to indirect direct questions to gather further information: 'What games do you play? If ꞁhad a race in your class where will you come? Can you play like your friends or ꞁou get out of 'puff' and have to stop?' There is no point in asking, for example, ꞁ much exercise can you do?' The parent can then be asked to fill in any other ꞁant information or to correct any information they feel needs amending. At the ꞁof the consultation, make sure you let the child know – in simple language – ꞁt you would like them to do and thank them.

ꞁ will be marked down if you fail to engage with the child – always ꞁ to them first.

ꞁommunication station is not a knowledge testing exercise. You do not have to how much you know of a particular condition – it is about **how you engage the patient and their parent**, develop a two-way dialogue, elicit and ꞁss their concerns and give what information they need, in a language and ꞁer they can understand.

ꞁo establish what they know already, make a judgement of their level ꞁderstanding and pitch your message appropriately. One approach is to ꞁhat they do for a living and the language of your answers could then be ꞁent, though not the content, if you were speaking to a cleaner, for example, ꞁr than a physics teacher in secondary school. My suggestion would be to ꞁas if you are talking to a 10-year-old and then adjust your replies on the ꞁack and questions you get in response.

ꞁfore, in a successful DCH communication exercise you will:

ꞁiliarise yourself with the background of a case

ꞁꞁe some knowledge of management options

ꞁroduce yourself

ꞁck how the 'patient' would like to be addressed

ꞁke eye contact

- Ask them to summarise what they have understood and wh:
- Discuss follow-up:
  - next appointment
  - plan for unexpected outcomes.

How much information should be given to a patient is a longst
It is now agreed, however, that all relevant facts should be giv
reassuring and encouraging, and this will also ensure bett
co-operation with treatment. This should include what investi
what will be involved, what they might show, what the diagnc
the treatment may be and the likely outcome.

Good communication requires that patient's concerns are tak
explored, and that at the conclusion of the meeting the patiei
the nature of the diagnosis, treatment and prognosis of their

**In the context of the communication station, you should
points that need to be discussed and it will be useful to :
that come to mind while waiting outside the room read:**

Remember, you do not have to cover everything that you knc
about the style of giving information and ensuring the infor
I have seen candidates in the heat of the examination come
then continue speaking, without actively looking at the pati
response until they have said all they can remember. The p:
usually have switched off after the first 30 seconds, and so

It is best to give information in small, bite-sized chunks an
more than 30 seconds without:

- getting a response from the patient, be it verbal or nonv
- asking them to repeat what they have understood.

After the bell, it is best to summarise, for example: 'So we
c, and we have agreed x, y and z. We will meet again for a

To conclude, communication is fundamental to our interac
and essential in our relationships with patients. We use a:
of communication discussed earlier, often without being a:
from one to the other seamlessly.

You should use spoken words most of the time but be awa
usefulness of written words and diagrams as these are al
getting your message across.

P:

Ou
wo
the
im
po:
wi
a q
yes
anc
you
do :
'Ho
rele
end
wha

You
spe

The
sho
wit
add:
man

Try
of ur
ask
diffe:
rathe
start
feedl

Ther

- fa
- ha
- in
- ch
- m:

- Ask them to summarise what they have understood and what they will do.
- Discuss follow-up:
  - next appointment
  - plan for unexpected outcomes.

How much information should be given to a patient is a longstanding dilemma. It is now agreed, however, that all relevant facts should be given, which should be **reassuring and encouraging**, and this will also ensure better acceptance of and co-operation with treatment. This should include what investigations are needed, what will be involved, what they might show, what the diagnosis might be, what the treatment may be and the likely outcome.

Good communication requires that patient's concerns are taken, understood and explored, and that at the conclusion of the meeting the patient understands about the nature of the diagnosis, treatment and prognosis of their illness.

In the context of the communication station, you should make a list of the points that need to be discussed and it will be useful to make a list of ideas that come to mind while waiting outside the room reading the script.

Remember, you do not have to cover everything that you know on a topic; it is about the style of giving information and ensuring the information is understood. I have seen candidates in the heat of the examination come in, sit down and then continue speaking, without actively looking at the patient/role-player for a response until they have said all they can remember. The patient/role-player will usually have switched off after the first 30 seconds, and so will the examiner.

It is best to give information in small, bite-sized chunks and to **NOT speak for more than 30 seconds** without:

- getting a response from the patient, be it verbal or nonverbal

- asking them to repeat what they have understood.

After the bell, it is best to summarise, for example: 'So we have discussed a, b and c, and we have agreed x, y and z. We will meet again for a follow up on…'.

To conclude, communication is fundamental to our interaction with other people, and essential in our relationships with patients. We use all of the various methods of communication discussed earlier, often without being aware of it, and we move from one to the other seamlessly.

You should use spoken words most of the time but be aware of the relevance and usefulness of written words and diagrams as these are also very effective ways of getting your message across.

Paediatric three-way consultation

Our patients are children, but it will primarily be their parents who will be anxious, worried, and who will ask most of the questions. We therefore have to develop the skills to be able to engage **both** child and parent appropriately. It is always important to interact with the child and include them in the discussion as much as possible. **Ignore the child at your peril**. If a child is present, start by interacting with them using an opening, welcoming remark or introducing yourself and asking a question they should be able to answer, such as 'What did you do at school yesterday?' or 'What do you like best at school?' You can then move on to indirect and direct questions to gather further information: 'What games do you play? If you had a race in your class where will you come? Can you play like your friends or do you get out of 'puff' and have to stop?' There is no point in asking, for example, 'How much exercise can you do?' The parent can then be asked to fill in any other relevant information or to correct any information they feel needs amending. At the end of the consultation, make sure you let the child know – in simple language – what you would like them to do and thank them.

You will be marked down if you fail to engage with the child – always speak to them first.

The communication station is not a knowledge testing exercise. You do not have to show how much you know of a particular condition – it is about **how you engage with the patient and their parent**, develop a two-way dialogue, elicit and address their concerns and give what information they need, in a language and manner they can understand.

Try to establish what they know already, make a judgement of their level of understanding and pitch your message appropriately. One approach is to ask what they do for a living and the language of your answers could then be different, though not the content, if you were speaking to a cleaner, for example, rather than a physics teacher in secondary school. My suggestion would be to start as if you are talking to a 10-year-old and then adjust your replies on the feedback and questions you get in response.

Therefore, in a successful DCH communication exercise you will:

- familiarise yourself with the background of a case
- have some knowledge of management options
- introduce yourself
- check how the 'patient' would like to be addressed
- make eye contact

- confirm the identity of the person and cross-check their relationship with the child
- confirm the task set and ask if anything else is required
- explain in small, bite-sized bits of information (30 second)
- use pauses and silence to emphasise information
- regularly check the message is being understood
- look out for verbal and nonverbal cues
- ask them to repeat what they have understood
- offer to provide information in the form of leaflets
- finish and summarise at the end
- be sensitive and do not interrupt
- try to remain positive
- make a safety net – arrange to review if required.

Final preparation for the communication station: the nuts and bolts

Remember, the exam situation is very artificial. It is a 'play' or 'drama', with each member having a designated role. You, the examiner, the patient or role-player, act to a script with some free play.

As you work through the scenarios in this book, it is a good idea to record your interactions with a camera or your mobile phone, with 'mock patients' or 'students' or colleagues. This will give you a very important opportunity to critically review and improve your performance. On reviewing the footage, preferably in a small group, you will notice the difference in one another's styles and can consider the impact of different approaches. This will help you adapt, modify and improve your own technique.

This will improve with practice.

We now have some typical communications you might come across in the DCH examination. Do not just read them as a story – practise with a friend or on your own but then use a camera or smart phone to record your performance to be reviewed with a critical eye. This approach can be used through all the scenarios in the book.

References

Makoul G (2001) Essential elements of communication in medical encounters: the kalamazoo consensus statement. *Academic Medicine* **76** (4) 390–3.

Roter D & Larson S (2002) The Roter interaction analysis system (RIAS): utility and flexibility for analysis of medical interactions. *Patient education and counselling* **46** (4) 243–51.

Communication station: case 1

Diagnosis of asthma

Information given to the candidate

You are a GP registrar.

You are seeing Sol's mother after making a diagnosis of asthma. Sol is four years old.

Your task

Discuss and explain the management of Sol's condition with his mother, Mrs Rosenberg.

You are not expected to gather any further medical history but answer any queries that may arise during the discussion.

You have six minutes to complete the station; a warning bell will be given at five minutes.

Information available to role-player

- You are Elaine Rosenberg, and you would like to be called Elaine.
- You had asthma as a child.
- Sol has had two admissions to the hospital in the first two years of life with breathing difficulties.
- Now he has been coughing at night and gets tired easily when playing.
- He has eczema, for which he is on treatment.

Concerns you have and information you want to find out

- What medications will Sol need?
- For how long and will he grow out of it?
- You are concerned about using steroids.
- How is the doctor going to monitor him?
- Where can you get more information?
- Is there an asthma nurse who can help you?
- What should you do if he worsens again?

What is expected from the candidate

The candidate should:

- introduce themself to Mrs Rosenberg and ask about Sol's well-being
- take a lead from how she replies as to how to address her
- refer to the role-player as 'Elaine', and not as mum or mother
- address the child by his name
- explain and agree the agenda for the clinical discussion
- explain the diagnostic criteria for asthma and simple pathophysiology
- explain that peak flow and spirometry may be used in the future to assess progression
- use British Thoracic Society (BTS) guidelines for management
- arrange follow-up with a specialist asthma nurse as available
- give a clear management plan and follow-up plans
- not gather further history or unnecessary information
- summarise the discussion and address any other concerns raised by Sol's mother
- frequently check mother's understanding
- avoid monologues – speak for no more than 30 seconds before checking understanding or seeking any questions
- not use medical jargon.

Further information

Asthma is a very common condition usually presenting in children with a strong family history of atopy. Children often present with a nocturnal and exercise induced cough.

Diagnosis and management guidelines of the British Thoracic Society can be found at: https://www.brit-thoracic.org.uk/document-library/clinical-information/asthma/btssign-guideline-on-the-management-of-asthma/

For your notes and thoughts

Communication station: case 2

Febrile convulsion

Information given to the candidate

You are a GP registrar.

You are visiting Mark, a 15-month-old boy who has had a generalised convulsion lasting 30 seconds. He has been unwell for the last two days with coryzal symptoms and now feels hot, but is alert and looking around appropriately.

Your task

Discuss with Andrew, his father, who is very concerned.

You are not expected to gather any further medical history but answer any queries that may arise during the discussion.

You have six minutes to complete the station; a warning bell will be given at five minutes.

Information available to role-player

You are Andrew, a 21-year-old builder, and Mark is your first child. Mark's mother is away for a few days visiting family:

- Mark has been unwell for the past two days with what you thought was a cold. You have had a cold yourself.
- He has been having high temperatures and you have been giving him paracetamol as advised by the doctor.
- Mark was sleeping with you when you woke up and noticed him to be shaking and he felt very hot to touch.
- You thought he was going to die and you rang 999 but by the time the ambulance crew came he was fine and that's why they called the doctor.

Concerns you have and information you want to find out

- Why did it happen?
- Does he have epilepsy?
- Is he going to have brain damage?
- Could it happen again?

What is expected from the candidate

The candidate should:

- introduce themself to Andrew and ask about Mark's well-being
- take a lead from how he replies as to how to address him
- refer to the role-player as 'Andrew' and not as dad or father
- address the child by his name
- explain and agree the agenda for the clinical discussion
- reassure Andrew that Mark is not going to die
- explain that there is no permanent damage
- explain about febrile convulsions
- give Andrew access to NHS information website
- establish safety nets and arrange to see Mark again
- give a clear management plan and follow-up plans
- not gather further history or unnecessary information
- summarise the discussion and address any other concerns raised by Andrew
- frequently check Andrew's understanding
- avoid monologues – speak for no more than 30 seconds before checking understanding or seeking any questions
- not use medical jargon.

Further information

- A febrile seizure/febrile convulsion occurs with a fever.
- It may be the first indication to parents that a child is unwell.
- It is a relatively common childhood condition.
- During most seizures, the child's body becomes stiff, they lose consciousness and their arms and legs jerk. Some children may wet themselves.
- It may be tonic or tonic-clonic.
- Parents find the experience very frightening and often say they thought the child was going to die.
- Most febrile seizures are harmless and do not pose a threat to a child's health.
- They can recur in about one-third of children during subsequent febrile illnesses.
- General advice is to keep the child cool and give antipyretics if required. **Note:** antipyretics do not prevent febrile convulsions.
- During a fit, parents should observe basic life-support skills. These should be demonstrated to parents before discharging a child home.
- Long-term epilepsy incidence is the same as for general population, around one per cent.

For more information, visit: http://www.nhs.uk/Conditions/Febrile-convulsions/Pages/Introduction.aspx

For your notes and thoughts

Communication station: case 3

Non-blanching rash

Information given to the candidate

You are a GP.

Saira, a two-year-old, is brought to the surgery by her mother who has noticed a rash on her abdomen and a 24-hour history of fever and feeling 'grizzly'.

On examination, you find the rash to be purpuric and consider meningococcal sepsis.

Your task

Explain your management plan to Saira's mother.

You are not expected to gather any further medical history but answer any queries that may arise during the discussion.

You have six minutes to complete the station; a warning bell will be given at five minutes.

Information available to role-player
- You are Saira's mother, Anjum Chaudhry, and you like to be referred to as Anjie.
- Saira has been unwell like this before and you are expecting the doctor to reassure you.
- Her friends have had rashes before.
- You are surprised at the seriousness of the situation.
- You become worried when they tell you about the urgent need to go to hospital.

Concerns you have and information you want to find out
- What does this rash mean and why is it so serious?
- What is the doctor going to do about it?
- Is her life in danger?
- What will they do with her in the hospital?
- What about Iqbal, her seven-year-old brother at home?

What is expected from the candidate

The candidate should:

- introduce themself to Anjie and asks about Saira's well-being
- take a lead from how she replies as to how to address her
- refer to the role-player as 'Anjie' and not as mum or mother
- address the child by her name
- explain and agree the agenda for the clinic discussion
- arrange to give intramuscular penicillin
- contact the local paediatric unit and arrange an urgent admission
- arrange transport via ambulance and not personal transport
- give an idea of the likely management in hospital (admission, IV antibiotics, IV fluids)
- ask about contacts and offer to arrange antibiotic prophylaxis for Iqbal and Anjie
- not gather further history or unnecessary information
- summarise the discussion and address any other concerns raised by Saira's mother
- frequently check Anjie's understanding
- avoid monologues – speak for no more than 30 seconds before checking understanding or seeking any questions
- not use medical jargon.

Further information

There is usually a rapid deterioration in a child's condition with meningococcal sepsis, and it is therefore important to administer the initial dose of intramuscular antibiotics rapidly. Although mortality is high, it can be improved with prompt treatment.

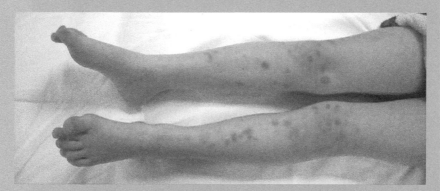

Rash of meningococcal sepsis can be erythematous and blanching early on in the illness and later turns pupuric.

For more information, visit: www.nlm.nih.gov/medlineplus/ency/article/001349.htm or www.nice.org.uk/nicemedia/live/13027/49339/49339.pdf

For your notes and thoughts

Communication station: case 4

Angry mother unhappy with 'out of hours' review

Information given to the candidate

You are a GP.

You are seeing Elsie, the mother of three-year-old Daisy. Daisy has been complaining of abdominal pain and was seen by the out of hours doctor.

The child was found to be well with a mild upper respiratory tract infection (URTI). You confirm the diagnosis.

Your task

Discuss the mother's concerns.

You are not expected to gather any further medical history but answer any queries that may arise during the discussion.

You have six minutes to complete the station; a warning bell will be given at five minutes.

Information available to the role-player

- You are Elsie, a 25 year-old-health care assistant.
- You like to be called Elsie.
- You think your daughter has been off-colour for five days.
- You called the doctor last night as she was complaining of severe tummy pain.
- The doctor rushed the examination and seemed to be in a hurry.
- You think your daughter may have appendicitis.
- He said there was nothing seriously wrong with Daisy, though you disagree.
- You felt he didn't take you seriously and have come for a second opinion.

What is expected from the candidate

The candidate should:

- introduce themself to Elsie and ask about Daisy's well-being
- take a lead from how she replies as to how to address her
- refer to the role-player as 'Elsie' and not as mum or mother
- address the child by her name
- explains and agree the agenda for the clinical discussion
- explore Elsie's ideas, concerns and expectations
- explain the findings to Elsie and reassure her that Daisy does not have a serious condition, eg. appendicitis
- not undermine the clinical assessment and advice of the out of hours doctor
- explain that Daisy is likely to grow out of this and has a good prognosis
- give a clear management plan and follow-up plans
- not gather further history or unnecessary information
- summarise the discussion and address any other concerns raised by Daisy's mother
- frequently check mother's understanding
- avoid monologues – speak for no more than 30 seconds before checking understanding or seeking any questions
- not use medical jargon.

Further information

Out of hours is an 'on call' service that provides emergency consultations.

Communication with parents/carers is very important and it is important to consider it under the following well-documented and researched tool for communication – ICE:

I – Ideas.

C – Concerns.

E – Expectations.

Give parents enough time to express their concerns and do not interrupt. They will rarely speak for more than one minute.

Your answers should be in bite-sized chunks and you should not speak for more than 30 seconds.

For your notes and thoughts

Communication station: case 5

Vaccination

Information given to the candidate

You are a GP registrar.

Sophia has come to discuss vaccinations for her newborn son, William, who is two weeks old. She also has an older daughter Mary, three, who has not been immunised.

She has heard of a measles epidemic in another part of the country.

Your task

Discuss Sophia's concerns and advise her on current immunisation policy.

You are not expected to gather any further medical history but answer any queries that may arise during the discussion.

You have six minutes to complete the station; a warning bell will be given at five minutes.

Information available to role-player

- You are Sophia Jones and you like to be referred to as Sophia.
- William and Mary are both well.
- You have heard on the news of a measles outbreak and are surprised at the seriousness of the situation.
- You became worried when you heard that some children have died following the infection.
- You heard that 'jabs' can cause brain damage, hence you did not get Mary immunised.
- You do not want your children to catch the illness and die.

Concerns you have and information you want to find out

- Will it help if you keep them indoors?
- If you want to give the vaccinations, what does it involve?

What is expected from the candidate

The candidate should:

- introduce themself to Sophia and ask about Mary and William's well-being
- take a lead from how she replies as to how to address her
- refer to the role-player as 'Sophia' and not as mum or mother
- address the children by their names
- explain and agree the agenda for the clinic discussion
- give a brief explanation of the immunisation programme
- put the risks and side effects in perspective
- arrange for an information leaflet for Sophia to take and read
- recommend that Mary should also be immunised
- arrange to meet the family again in order to discuss any concerns and arrange dates for vaccinations
- not gather further history or unnecessary information
- summarise the discussion and address any other concerns raised by Sophia
- frequently check Sophia's understanding
- avoid monologues – speak for no more than 30 seconds before checking understanding or seeking any questions
- not use medical jargon.

Further information

Vaccinations are important to prevent communicable diseases. All candidates should be familiar with the concept of herd immunity.

Egg allergy is NOT a contraindication to measles vaccination.

For more information, visit: www.nhs.uk/vaccinations

For your notes and thoughts

Communication station: case 6

Chickenpox

Information given to the candidate

You are a GP.

You see Emily, a 25-year-old who is 12 weeks pregnant. She has come to the surgery with her 18-month-old son, John, who has been unwell for three days with UTRI like symptoms and has now come out in a rash with a few vesicles.

You diagnose John with chickenpox.

Your task

Discuss management of the condition with Emily.

You are not expected to gather any further medical history but answer any queries that may arise during the discussion.

You have six minutes to complete the station; a warning bell will be given at five minutes.

Information available to role-player

- You are Emily, 25 years old, and you have come to see your GP.
- You prefer to be called Emily.
- You are 12 weeks pregnant.
- Your son, John, has been unwell for three days and now has come out in a rash.
- You are very worried by the information you have read on the web.
- You have not had chickenpox as far as you can remember but you are not sure.
- A blood test may be advised to detect antibodies to see if you are immune.
- About one in 10 pregnant women has not previously had chickenpox and is therefore not immune.
- If you are not immune you can be given treatment which may reduce the risk to you and your baby.

 Diploma in Child Health: Volume 1 © Pavilion Publishing and Media Ltd and its licensors 2014.

What is expected from the candidate

The candidate should:

- introduce themself to Emily and ask about John's well-being
- take a lead from how she replies as to how to address her
- refer to the role-player as 'Emily' and not as mum or mother
- address the child by his name
- explain and agree the agenda for the clinic discussion
- give a brief outline of the risks of chickenpox
- explain that chickenpox has a good outcome in the majority of cases, that it is self-limiting
- advise to encourage oral fluids and give antipyretics
- offer blood tests to check Emily's immune status. Give clear management and follow-up plans
- not gather further history or unnecessary information
- summarise the discussion and address any other concerns raised by John's mother
- frequently check Emily's understanding
- avoid monologues – speak for no more than 30 seconds before checking understanding or seeking any questions
- not use medical jargon.

Further information

Approximately three in 1,000 pregnant women develop chickenpox. Chickenpox during pregnancy can cause complications both for the pregnant woman and the foetus. However, the risk of complications is low.

A person may be susceptible if:

- they are in the same room as someone with chickenpox for more than 15 minutes
- they have any face-to-face contact with someone with chickenpox.

Chickenpox is infectious from two days before the rash first appears until all the spots have crusted over, which is usually about five days after the onset of the rash. Immunoglobulin can be given to alter the course of disease.

Complications

For the mother:

Chickenpox is typically an unpleasant illness, and more severe than in children. Complications can include:

- Pneumonia.
- Encephalitis, however this is rare.
- Others:
  - myocarditis
  - glomerulonephritis
  - appendicitis, hepatitis
  - pancreatitis
  - Henoch-Schönlein purpura
  - arthritis
  - uveitis.

For the foetus:

- May develop fetal varicella syndrome (FVS) causing congenital abnormalities.
- In the first 12 weeks of pregnancy there is a 1 in 200 chance of the baby developing FVS.
- Between 13 and 20 weeks of pregnancy there is a 1 in 50 chance of the baby developing FVS.
- After 20 weeks the risk of the baby developing FVS is very low.
- There have been no reported cases in women who developed chickenpox after 28 weeks.

For the newborn baby:

The baby may develop severe chickenpox and will need treatment if a mother gets chickenpox:

- around the time of the birth and the baby is born within seven days of the mother developing chickenpox.
- up to seven days after giving birth.

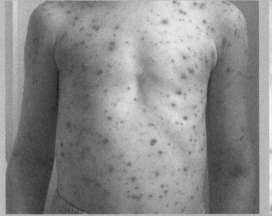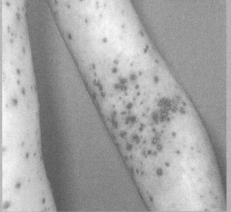

Child with typical chickenpox rash, some crusting.

For more information, see:
http://www.nhs.uk/chq/Pages/1109.aspx?CategoryID=54&SubCategoryID=137#close
http://www.patient.co.uk/health/Chickenpox-Contact-and-Pregnancy

For your notes and thoughts

Communication station: case 7

Traffic light system – with trainee

Information given to the candidate

You are a GP.

Raj, your GP trainee ST1, comes to you for clarification on the 'traffic light system' (TLS), which he has been asked to use by the practice nurse.

Your task

Please discuss the 'traffic light system' and address his queries.

You are not expected to gather unnecessary information but answer any queries that may arise during the discussion.

You have six minutes to complete the station; a warning bell will be given at five minutes.

Information available to role-player

You are Raj, an ST1 in general practice. This is your first general practice placement. A practice nurse has mentioned the traffic light system to assess children. You would like to know the following:

- What is TLS?
- How is it used?
- How is it different from other clinical evaluations that you use?

If the candidate asks 'What do you know about it or have you read anything on it?' you can lead in with the following, or if the candidate does not know anything about the topic – you can help:

- It is used to assess children.
- I have done some reading on it.
- It is used to identify likelihood of serious illness.
- Green – Amber – Red.

- It is based on the following factors:
  - colour
  - activity
  - respiratory status
  - hydration
  - other symptoms and signs.

What is expected from the candidate

The candidate should:

- introduce themself to the trainee and ask about their well-being
- take a lead from how he replies as to how to address him
- refer to the role-player as 'Raj'
- explain and agree the agenda for the meeting and discussion
- if he does not know much about the topic, ask the trainee:
  - what he does know about the topic
  - whether he has done any reading on it
- arrange to meet again and discuss the topic in few days
- avoid monologue – speak for no for more than 30 seconds before checking understanding or seeking any questions
- not use complicated medical jargon.

Further information

The traffic light system is a guideline used to identify serious illness in a febrile child. It offers evidence-based advice on the care of young children with feverish illnesses.

A recent review of evidence suggests that it is more useful when combined with a bedside urine analysis.

For more information and to see an example of the traffic light table, visit: http://guidance.nice.org.uk/CG160

For your notes and thoughts

Communication station: case 8

Chest pain

Information given to the candidate

You are the paediatric SHO.

You have seen Michael, a nine-year-old boy, with his mother Samantha, who is very concerned. Michael has complained of central chest pains a few times a day, lasting a few seconds, for the past two weeks. It can happen at rest or while playing. His grandfather recently had a myocardial infarction. An ECG has been done and is normal.

In your opinion the pain is non-cardiac and but may be due to reflux or muscle 'stitch'.

Your task

Discuss your proposed management plan with Michael's mother.

You are not expected to gather any further medical history, but answer any queries that may arise during the discussion.

You have six minutes to complete the station; a warning bell will be given at five minutes.

Information available to role-player

You are Samantha and you have come with Michael, who is nine years old:

- He has complained of chest pains for two weeks.
- Pain is in the middle of his chest and lasts few seconds a time.
- It can happen either when he is resting or playing.
- He is not bothered by the pain.

Concerns you have and information you want to find out

- You are very concerned as your father has recently had a heart attack.
- You have checked on the internet and found that chest pain can be very serious.
- You want tests done on Michael.
- You want definite answers.
- If the doctor refuses any tests you can get angry.
- Show appropriate emotions.

What is expected from the candidate

The candidate should:
- introduce themself to Samantha and ask about Michael's well-being
- take a lead from how she replies as to how to address her
- refer to role-player as 'Samantha' and not as mum or mother
- address the child by his name
- explain and agree the agenda for the clinical discussion
- acknowledge Samantha's concerns
- explain that the pain does not have a serious cause
- explain that there is no need for further tests and that the ECG was normal
- explain that he is likely to grow out of this and has a good prognosis
- give the option of using antacid in case it is due to reflux, or paracetamol if the pain is prolonged
- give clear management and follow-up plans
- not gather further history or unnecessary information
- summarise the discussion and address any other concerns raised by Michael's mother
- frequently checks Samantha's understanding
- avoid monologues – speak for no more than 30 seconds before checking understanding or seeking any questions
- not use medical jargon.

Further information

Paediatric chest pain is mostly non-cardiac in origin, benign and self-limiting in the majority of cases. It may be due to:
- Structural abnormality of chest organs
- Pneumothorax
- Pneumonia
- Asthma
- Functional abnormality of the rib cage/spine/musculoskeletal:
  - costochondritis/Tietz syndrome
  - injury to muscles and bones
  - non-specific or idiopathic chest wall pain
  - sickle cell crisis
  - spinal nerve root compression.

- Referred from organs in the abdomen:
  - gastro-oesophageal reflux
  - oesophagitis.

With cardiac chest pain, although not common, the following should be kept in mind:

- Pericarditis.
- Coronary artery abnormalities – very rare and presents in neonatal period.

Other possible causes include:

- stress and anxiety
- herpes zoster infection.

For more information, see:

http://pedsinreview.aappublications.org/content/31/1/e1.full

http://www.rightdiagnosis.com/sym/chest_pain_in_children.htm

http://ic.steadyhealth.com/chest_pain_in_children.html

For your notes and thoughts

Communication station: case 9

Triple stool infection

Information given to the candidate

You are a GP.

Mrs Smith comes to see you with her daughter, Claire, who is three years old. Claire has loose stools and abdominal pain. There are pieces of undigested food in the stools. Her mother had her stools analysed at a private clinic. She brings a report showing bacterial, fungal and protozoal organisms found on the stool sample. She demands medications for the three infections.

Your task

Discuss your management plan with Mrs Smith.

You are not expected to gather any further medical history, but answer any queries that may arise during the discussion.

You have six minutes to complete the station; a warning bell will be given at five minutes.

Information available to the role-player

- You are the mother of Claire and you have come to see your GP to discuss your daughter's results from a private clinic.
- You would like to be called Jane.

Concerns you have and information you want to find out

- Why does Claire have so many 'bugs' in her stools?
- Where did she get them?
- Why were they not picked up previously?
- Why are you not treating them?
- If the doctor does not treat them, what are they going to do?
- What about her discomfort?
- When will she get better?
- Can she go to play group?

What is expected from the candidate

The candidate should:

- introduce themself to Jane and ask about Claire's well-being
- take a lead from how she replies as to how to address her
- refer to the role-player as 'Claire' and not as mum or mother
- address the child by her name
- explain and agree the agenda for the discussion
- discuss the results from the private clinic
- reassure Jane that Claire is 'normal'
- explain that tests will be repeated for confirmation, and if anything is found to be 'abnormal' then act accordingly
- not agree to prescribe antibiotics/medication
- explain that it is likely to be toddler diarrhoea
- normalise the condition and put the symptoms in perspective
- explain that Claire is likely to grow out of this and has a good prognosis
- give a clear management plan and follow-up plans
- not gather further history or unnecessary information
- summarise the discussion and address any other concerns raised by Claire's mother
- frequently check Jane's understanding
- avoid monologues – speak for no more than 30 seconds before checking understanding or seeking any questions
- not use medical jargon.

Further information

Toddler diarrhoea

Toddler diarrhoea is considered in children:

- who are perfectly healthy and are growing normally
- aged between one and five years
- who pass frequent, smelly, loose stools
- whose stools contain recognisable foods, such as carrots and peas.

It is more common in boys than girls.

Toddler diarrhoea is not serious and will improve by the time children are about five years old.

There are about 100 trillion micro-organisms in the intestine, the majority of which are commensals and cause no harm to the body.

Diarrhoea and vomiting in children

Rota virus is a common cause of vomiting and diarrhoea in children.

With formula-fed babies, sterilisation of bottles is extremely important.

It is important to watch for signs of dehydration:

- Lethargy.
- Irritability.
- Dry mouth.
- Loose, pale or mottled skin.
- Sunken eyes and fontanelle.

General advice:

- Give extra fluids. Give the baby oral rehydration fluids in between feeds or after each watery stool.
- Use oral rehydration solution.
- Do not stop feeding the baby milk or dilute milk feeds. Give the extra fluid as an addition to milk.
- Ensure good hand hygiene practices are adhered to.

For more information, see:

http://www.nhs.uk/Conditions/pregnancy-and-baby/Pages/diarrhoea-vomiting-children.aspx

http://www.patient.co.uk/health/toddlers-diarrhoea

http://textbookofbacteriology.net/normalflora.html

http://pediatrics.about.com/od/weeklyquestion/a/05_tdl_diarrhea.htm

For your notes and thoughts

Communication station: case 10

Talking to a difficult colleague

Information given to the candidate

You are the GP registrar in the last month of your GP ST3. An F1 trainee posted to your surgery has been found to be altering the notes for patients he/she has not been directly involved with. The trainee has been noted to be late and has disappeared without leaving any information on three occasions.

Your task

Your supervisor has been called away to an emergency and has suggested that you go and speak to him/her. You are not expected to gather any further history.

You have six minutes to complete the station; a warning bell will be given at five minutes.

Information available to the role-player

You are an F1 trainee.

You had a difficult time in your last two postings as an F1 and concerns have been highlighted about your note keeping and data entry.

You have recently broken up with your partner but do not want to bring it up in your discussion.

You want to be perfect in your documentation and thereby make entries at a later point.

You know a couple of patients socially and felt that some entries made about their condition are not correct, hence you altered the notes for them.

You need to be told about GMC good medical practice.

You expect to be reported to your supervisor who is also worried about this.

What is expected from the candidate

The candidate should:

- introduce themself to the role-player and explain the agenda for the meeting
- exhibit empathy towards a struggling colleague and enquire about their well-being, but should not probe into their social/personal life
- acknowledge the F1 trainee's contribution to the team
- clearly enquire whether the F1 trainee made alterations to medical notes and their reasons for doing so for patients they haven't been directly involved with
- mention that medical notes are legal documents that should not be altered, and entries made later should be clearly dated and signed
- reassure them about the support to be provided
- not give false reassurance that the GP supervisor will not be informed as requested by the role-player
- mention that this is a learning opportunity for the trainee
- outline a clear plan for improvement
- mention GMC good medical practice
- summarise the discussion and offer to meet the trainee at a later date to find out about progress
- not use excessive medical jargon – however the candidate should use adequate medical terminology as they are speaking to a doctor – too much lay talk can be counterproductive.

Further information

Candidates are advised to read the GMC's *Good Medical Practice* guidance, available at: http://www.gmc-uk.org/guidance/good_medical_practice.asp (accessed February 2014).

For your notes and thoughts

Clinical examination station

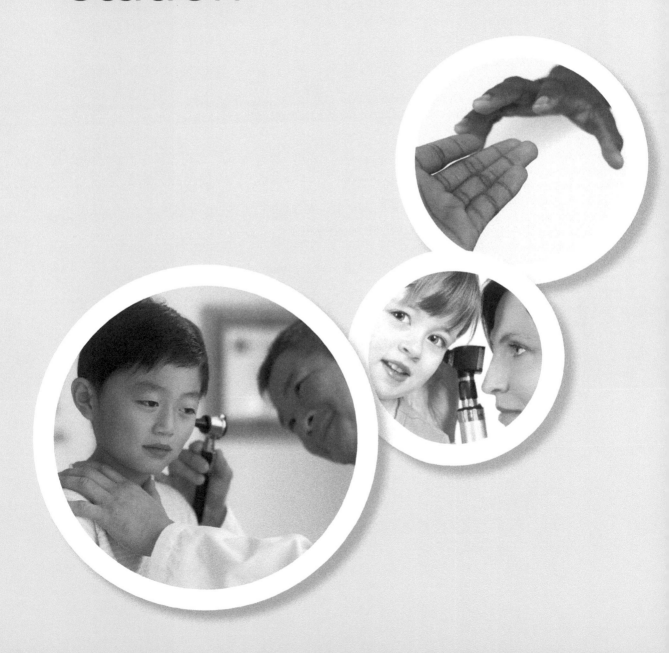

Clinical examination station

At this station you will meet real patients with a range of real conditions, who you will be expected to assess and diagnose. You could therefore encounter any clinical case, be it respiratory, cardiovascular, neurological, or any other, and you will need to be experienced at examining all systems and gathering your findings before giving a clear presentation to the examiner and engaging them in the all-important discussion.

The children who come to help with the examinations are not a special cohort, reserved for this purpose, but are patients you might encounter on the ward, in a hospital clinic or at the GP surgery. Most children you will assess in the examination will have taken part in the examinations before, and so they are usually quite conversant with the happenings of the examination. However, it is still vitally important to thank them for coming and helping, and to tell them what you will be doing or asking them to do in simple language that they can understand. At no point should you be 'rough' or 'rude' to the child. If you are having difficulty, do not force the child, let the examiner know what you would like to do – what you are looking for. Examiners have seen it all before and will guide you appropriately. With children, it is especially important to build a rapport and to be opportunistic in your examination technique.

A lot of information about a patient can be gathered by just observation:

■ What equipment is present in the room? A wheelchair or oxygen cylinder, for example.

■ What medications, such as inhalers or spacer devices, are in the room?

■ What is the child doing?

■ How does the child respond to his parents and strangers?

In real life, you decide on the 'system' to concentrate on using the information you have gathered during a general physical examination and the case history you have been given. In the examination, however, you will be given a brief introduction to the patient and directed to examine a particular system, be it cardiovascular, respiratory, abdominal etc. In a short space of time you have to build a rapport with the patient and their guardian, get their consent, do a general physical examination and then concentrate on the specified system, all within five or six minutes, as it is imperative you finish in time so as to have adequate room for discussion with the examiner, as that is where the marks will be. The examiner will observe you while you perform the physical examination, but will not disturb you unless you are rough with the child. They expect you to be systematic and proficient with your examination technique, brief and succinct in the presentation of your findings, and ready to discuss the differential diagnosis and management.

There are two options while examining: the first is to keep quiet, making a mental note of your findings and then presenting the findings at the end of your examination; the second is to declare your observations as you go along. Whichever approach you take, you will have to summarise at the end, giving your positive and negative findings. You should go with whichever you feel most comfortable, but clarify with the examiner which you will be doing. It is quite boring from the examiner's point to just watch in deadly silence as the candidate goes through the examination.

Your communication skills are vital to all the facets of your interaction with the patient, starting with first contact – first impressions count, after all.

After concluding your assessment of the child, your discussion with the examiner needs to be fluent and confident. Remember you are now in 'communication mode' and thus need to follow all the tips you will have learnt for the communication station.

To repeat: think before you start speaking; take a few seconds – you may think that an initial five or ten-second silence feels like an eternity, but a ten-second silence in the middle of a sentence, when the ideas just seem at the tip of the tongue but will not form, is a great deal more awkward and 'deafening'.

This emphasis on communication is not 'overkill', and the time you spend now on practising and improving this skill will help you more than anything else you may do so close to the exam.

You are not expected to know every rare syndrome for the DCH exam, however any good case with classical clinical signs might be selected for the exam. Even if you cannot arrive at a diagnosis, you should list out any abnormal features and try to formulate a possible differential diagnosis for them.

Using this chapter

In this chapter you will be presented with a series of patients and given some background information in the first box. In each case you are requested to perform a general examination and any other relevant examinations to reach a diagnosis and differential diagnosis.

The details of the examination are then explained in the second box, providing you with all the information you would be expected to have gathered if conducting a real examination.

In the DCH exam, you will then discuss your findings with the examiner. If you are working through this manual with a study partner, you should therefore ask them to role play the part of the examiner and they can use the 'findings' that are included in the third box. If you are working alone, write down your findings before referring to these 'answers'.

Practise them with your friends and colleagues, role play as appropriate and use every opportunity you get.

Clinical examination station: case 1

Osteogenesis imperfecta

Information given to the candidate

You enter the examination room and are introduced to the patient by the examiner.

Rachel, seven years old, is followed up by the orthopaedic and paediatric teams. She is admitted to the ward for her regular drug infusion.

Your task

You are requested to perform a general examination and any other relevant examinations to reach a diagnosis or differential diagnosis.

You are allowed to talk to the patient but are not allowed to ask any history unless allowed by the examiner.

You have nine minutes to complete the station; a warning bell will be given at seven minutes.

Examination

You introduce yourself to Rachel and her mother, and explain to them briefly what you will be doing and obtain a verbal consent to carry out the examination.

You explain that hand hygiene has been adhered to, or alternatively use alcohol gel in front of child and parent.

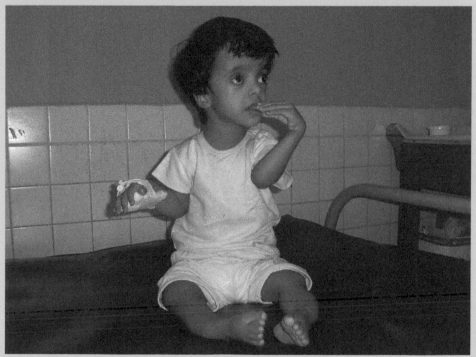

On general observation

- There is a walking aid close to the bed – an adapted tricycle.
- Rachel is comfortable and has an intravenous line in situ.
- She looks short for her age.

General physical and systemic examination

- Rachel has markedly deformed lower limbs, possibly due to repeated fractures.
- Blue sclera.
- Discoloured teeth.
- No widening of the wrists.
- No rickety rosary.
- No features suggestive of non-accidental injuries (NAI).

You turn to the examiner and summarise your findings.

Findings

You have examined seven-year-old Rachel, who is comfortable at rest. She seems to be short for her age but you would like to confirm this by plotting her on a growth chart. There is an adapted walking aid to support her mobility. The most striking feature is her deformed lower limbs, possibly due to fractures in the past. She also has blue-coloured sclera and discoloured dentition. There are no features suggestive of rickets or NAI.

You would like to ask her mother whether Rachel's hearing is affected.

You do not need to stop and can move on to your impression.

Your findings are consistent with osteogenesis imperfecta and her regular infusion must be bisphosphonates to increase bone density.

Be prepared to discuss osteogenesis imperfecta further. As this case is complex you are only expected to know the basic details.

What is expected from the candidate

The candidate should:

- introduce themself to Rachel and her mother
- request verbal consent to conduct the examination
- perform hand hygiene procedures
- keep the patient at ease throughout and give simple commands
- comment on the walking aid, growth and limb deformities
- identify that joint care from the paediatric and orthopaedic teams indicates chronic bone pathology
- exclude two other possible differentials (rickets and NAI), which will push the candidate for a clear pass.

Further information

Osteogenesis imperfecta is an inherited autosomal disorder, dominantly resulting in fragile bones due to defective and/or decreased type I collagen. It is usually classified into four types.

Type I: mildest and commonest (60%). Multiple fractures, triangular face, short stature, blue sclera, brittle and discoloured teeth (dentinogenesis imperfecta) and conductive deafness can occur.

Type II: Most severe and fatal. Neonates are severely affected with multiple fractures.

Type III: Similar to type I but severe as fractures are common at birth. Severe deafness can occur.

Type IV: Similar to type I. Teeth are defective but sclera colour is usually normal.

Affected children will receive multidisciplinary care, which includes supportive therapy (physical aids, splints) cyclical bisphosphonates (Pamidronate) to increase bone density and, rarely, surgery.

For more information, see:

http://www.nlm.nih.gov/medlineplus/osteogenesisimperfecta.html

http://www.oif.org/site/PageServer?pagename=fastfacts

For your notes and thoughts

Clinical examination station: case 2

Port-wine stain

Information given to the candidate

You enter the examination room and are introduced by the examiner to the patient. Two-year-old Sidney has come in for his routine six-month review.

Your task

You are requested to perform a general examination and any other relevant examinations to reach a diagnosis or differential diagnoses.

You are allowed to talk to the patient but are not allowed to ask any history unless allowed by the examiner.

You have nine minutes to complete the station; a warning bell will be given at seven minutes.

The examination

You introduce yourself to Sidney's mother, explain what you will be doing and obtain a verbal consent to carry out the investigation.

You explain that hand hygiene has been adhered to, or alternatively use alcohol gel in front of child and parent.

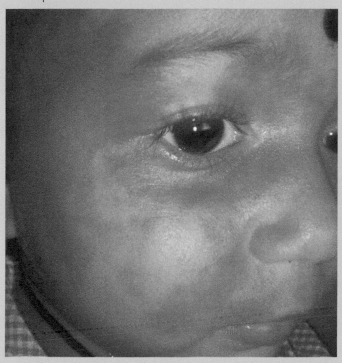

On general observation

- Sidney looks comfortable and well.
- His growth seems to be age appropriate but you would like to plot him on a growth chart.

General physical and systemic examination

- Sidney has an erythematous macular lesion over the face – distributed on the right side of the face involving the forehead, upper eyelid, upper lip and the cheek. It is clearly demarcated from the surrounding normal skin. No ulceration or changes to the overlying skin is noted.
- No other skin lesions noted.
- His gait is normal
- The appearance of the skin lesion is not suggestive of infantile haemangioma.

You turn to the examiner and summarise your findings.

Findings

You have examined two-year-old Sidney who is looking well and comfortable. He has a right-sided erythematous macular facial lesion involving the trigeminal nerve distribution. There are no other obvious skin lesions seen and his systemic examination is unremarkable.

You would like to ask his mother (if allowed by he examiner):

- whether the skin lesion was present from birth, whether it spread or if it has remained the same size
- if Sidney has ever had any seizures
- if his vision has been assessed.

You do not need to stop and can move on to your impression.

Your findings are consistent of right-sided port-wine stain. You would like to assess him further for any associations, such as Sturge-Weber syndrome.

What is expected from the candidate

The candidate should:

- introduce themself to Sidney and his mother
- request verbal consent to perform the examination
- perform hand hygiene procedures or explain that these have been carried out
- follow a logical sequence to examination
- keep the patient at ease and give easy to understand commands
- explain in detail about the skin lesion (distribution, colour, any changes)
- investigate whether there are any other associated skin lesions
- appreciate the port-wine stain does not appear like a typical haemagioma
- discuss the associated features of sturge-weber syndrome.

Further information

Port-wine stain (PWS)

PWS is always present from birth and is due to malformation of blood vessels. The colour darkens with age from an initial red/pink.

It can be associated with:

- glaucoma – same side of the skin lesion
- Sturge-Weber syndrome (SWS):
  - Port-wine stain commonly involving the ophthalmic (V1) and maxillary (V2) area of trigeminal nerve.

- Hemiparesis.
- Glaucoma.
- Learning disabilities.
- Focal seizures and sometimes generalised epilepsy and infantile spasms can occur. Focal seizures are on the same side to skin lesion.

Intracranial calcifications can be seen in skull x-ray or CT scan.

Management:
- For PWS – laser therapy.
- For SWS:
  - Anticonvulsants.
  - Intra-occular pressure monitoring.
  - Epilepsy surgery for resistant cases.

Infantile haemangiomas

Infantile haemangiomas are benign and are rarely present at birth. They appear within the first few weeks of life, initially enlarge and then, due to lack of blood supply, gradually decrease in size and disappear by five years of age.

There are two main types:
- Strawberry haemangioma – superficial and bright red.
- Cavernous haemangioma – deep and bluish.

Complications can include:
- ulceration
- bleeding
- breathing difficulties
- swallowing difficulties
- visual compromise.

Treatments include:
- oral propranolol for strawberry haemangioma
- laser therapy
- intra-lesional steroid injection.

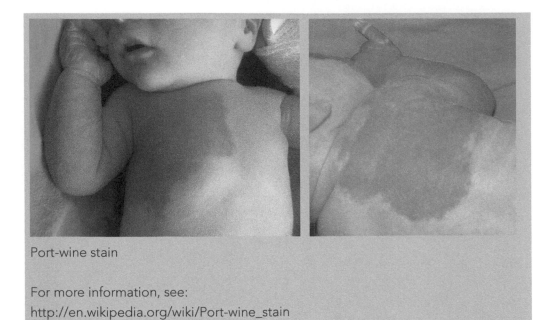

Port-wine stain

For more information, see:

http://en.wikipedia.org/wiki/Port-wine_stain

http://www.gosh.nhs.uk/medical-conditions/search-for-medical-conditions/port-wine-stain/port-wine-stain-information/

For your notes and thoughts

Clinical examination station: case 3

Central sternotomy scar

Information given to the candidate

You enter the examination room and are introduced to the patient by the examiner. George, seven years old, is sitting on a chair with his mother.

George has come for a routine check up. He looks well and is wearing shorts.

Your task

Perform a cardiovascular examination and any other relevant examinations to reach a diagnosis.

You are allowed to talk to the patient but are not allowed to ask any history unless the examiner says so.

You have nine minutes to complete the station; a warning bell will be given at seven minutes.

The examination

You introduce yourself to George and his mother, explain to them what you will be doing and obtain a verbal consent to perform the examination.

You explain that hand hygiene has been adhered to, or alternatively use alcohol gel in front of child and parent.

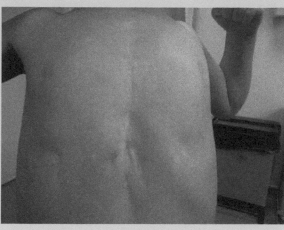

On general inspection:
- There are no medications or medical devices around.
- George is of average size and build.
- He is comfortable, pink and not in distress.
- Median sternotomy scar, normal skin colour, pale pink.
- Pectus excavatum.
- Two little scars in lower thoracic area.

General physical and systemic exam
- No clubbing.
- No cyanosis.
- Brachial/radials pulse equal, 80 min, regular.
- Central scar not tender.
- Precordium – no heave or thrill, apex 6th ICS and anterior axillary line.
- Heart sounds: clicky noise heard, maximal in upper right sternal area.
- Pan systolic murmur 3/6 at lower left sternal area.
- No murmur heard at back.
- Femoral pulse is easily palpable.

You may be invited by the examiner to ask George or his mother a question. You can use this opportunity to ask what his surgery was for.

You turn to the examiner and summarise your findings.

Findings

You have examined George, a seven-year-old boy. He is comfortable at rest. He is pink and seems an age-appropriate size but you would like to plot him on an appropriate chart. He had a median sternotomy scar, which is pale pink, and two smaller scars in the lower thoracic/upper abdominal area. He has no clubbing or cyanosis.

He has a regular pulse: 80/min. Peripheral pulses are easily palpable with no radio-femoral delay. Precordium feels normal with no heaves or thrill. Apex is in anterior axillary line, in 6th ICS. On auscultation there is a loud systolic murmur grade 3/6, maximal in the lower left sternal area, heard all over precordium. His heart sounds are 'different'. They do not sound normal. They have a clicky character. There are no bruits or murmurs in the neck or the back.

You do not need to stop and can move on to your impression.

You think George is well. Your clinical findings suggest he has a ventricular septal defect (VSD). Displaced apex beat suggests cardiomegaly. He also has 'different' sounding heart sounds that you have not heard before but you think they could be due to a mechanical artificial valve.

It is not possible, generally, to comment on the cardiac abnormality/defect that was corrected by surgery, and you should mention this at the start of your discussion.

This patient has two abnormalities – a small VSD and a prosthetic aortic valve. He had critical aortic stenosis and had balloon dilatation soon after birth. This left him with a degree of stenosis and regurgitation of the aortic valve leading to cardiomegaly. The valve was replaced a few months ago, as the scar has not 'healed' fully and changed colour. This is also the origin of his 'clicky' heart sounds. The two small scars are likely to be due to post operative 'drains'. He is currently on anticoagulants.

The pan-systolic murmur is from the VSD. However, as the defect is small and not haemodynamically important, it has been left, even after surgery for aortic valve replacement. Small VSD can now be closed with devices implanted by trans-femoral catheter techniques – key-hole surgery.

In standard settings most doctors will not have had the opportunity to listen to a prosthetic valve, but they should be able to differentiate it from normal heart sounds. You should not be afraid to mention any findings that are NOT normal, even if you're unable to interpret them and explain what the pathology is.

What is expected from the candidate

The candidate should:

- introduce themself to George and his mother and request verbal consent to perform an examination
- perform hand hygiene procedures or explain that these have been carried out
- keep the patient at ease and give simple and easy to understand commands
- inspect and comment on observations
- comment on median scar; a good candidate will also mention its colour
- follow a logical sequence to cardiac examination
- auscultate the back and neck
- pick up 'different' heart sounds
- work through and conclude two different pathologies
- be able to correlate the findings and discuss aetiology and management
- offer to take blood pressure.

Further information

For more information, see:

http://www.nlm.nih.gov/medlineplus/ency/article/001099.htm

http://www.mayoclinic.com/health/ventricular-septal-defect/DS00614

For your notes and thoughts

Clinical examination station: case 4

Ventricular septal defect (VSD)

Information given to the candidate

You enter the examination room and the examiner introduces you to a five-year-old girl, Susan, and her mother, both sitting on a chair.

Susan has come for a check-up as she was noted to have a murmur during a school medical check. She looks well and is wearing shorts.

Your task

You are requested to perform a cardiovascular examination and any other relevant examinations to reach a diagnosis.

You are allowed to talk to the patient but are not allowed to ask any history unless allowed by the examiner.

You have nine minutes to complete the station; a warning bell will be given at seven minutes.

The examination

You introduce yourself to Susan and her mother, explain to them what you will be doing and obtain verbal consent to carry out the examination.

You explain that hand hygiene has been adhered to, or alternatively use alcohol gel in front of child and parent.

On general inspection

- There are no medications or medical devices around.
- Susan is of average size and build.
- She is comfortable, pink and not in distress.
- Her chest is normal in shape and she has a normal respiratory rate.
- No scars noted.

General physical and systemic examination

- No clubbing.
- No cyanosis.
- Brachial/radials pulse equal, 90/min, regular.
- Precordium – no heave or thrill, apex 5th ICS and mid clavicular line.
- Heart sounds: first and second normal.
- Harsh pan systolic murmur 3/6, maximal at lower left sternal area.
- Does not change with posture.
- No murmur heard at back.
- Femoral pulses easily palpable.

You turn to the examiner and summarise your findings.

Following this, be prepared to discuss your findings with the examiner as the case is simple and there should be ample time left until the bell rings.

Findings

You have examined Susan, a five-year-old girl. She is comfortable at rest. She is pink and seems appropriately grown but you would like to plot her on the appropriate growth chart. There are no scars. She has no clubbing or cyanosis. She has regular pulse, 90/min. Peripheral pulses are easily palpable with no radio-femoral delay. Precordium feels normal with no heaves or thrill. Apex is in mid-clavicular line, in 5th ICS. On auscultation there is a harsh pan-systolic murmur grade 3/6, maximal in the lower left sternal area. Her heart sounds, first and second, are heard and are normal. Second heart sound is not prominent. (*If you are not sure of split sounds then you should avoid commenting on it.*) There are no bruits or murmurs in the neck or the back.

You do not need to stop and can move on to your impression.

Susan is well. Your findings are consistent with a ventricular septal defect (VSD), however you would like to confirm this with further investigations. The most useful will be an echocardiogram, which will confirm anatomy and function, and to check for rhythm and electrical activity. If an echocardiogram is not available, suggest a CXR to look for cardiac size and pulmonary congestion.

What is expected from the candidate

The candidate should:

- introduce themself to Susan and her mother
- request verbal consent to perform the examination
- perform hand hygiene procedures or explain that these have been carried out
- follow a logical sequence to cardiac examination
- keep the patient at ease and give easy to understand commands
- inspect and comment on observations
- comment on the absence of scars
- auscultate precordium, neck and back
- feel for femoral pulse and offer to take blood pressure
- pick up normal heart sounds and murmur
- work through and evaluate different pathologies
- be able to correlate the findings and discuss aetiology and management.

Further information

In the current UK guidelines, prophylaxis against bacterial endocarditis is not recommended. It is important to mention this change in guidelines, however, as most parents will have been told differently in the past.

Medium to long-term outcome and need for follow up

A large number of VSDs close during childhood.

There are no restrictions on travel – however it should be mentioned on travel insurance.

If you are asked whether it could be anything else, do not take it as a trick – it may be that you are wrong and the examiner is trying to prompt you to reconsider your initial findings. If you are sure, then say you still think the most likely diagnosis is a VSD but you will consider a differential diagnosis, including:

- Pulmonary stenosis, which can be easily confused.
- Atrial septal defect – the murmur is softer in the upper left sternal border.

Never be dogmatic and assert that it is classic VSD, and that you are absolutely sure. This attitude, if you are wrong, suggests that you are inflexible and once you have made up your mind are not open to other suggestions. This can be disastrous as it demonstrates you may have difficulty revising your diagnosis and reconsidering thoughts.

Echocardiogram: picture of VSD on colour flow:

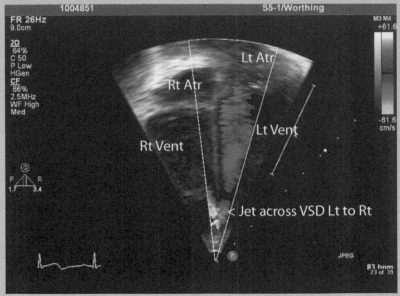

The picture shows a four chamber view of an echocardiogram. The colour flow doppler shows the jet of blood moving across the ventricular septal defect from left ventricle to right.

CXR: cardiomegaly with increased pulmonary markings suggestive of pulmonary congestion:

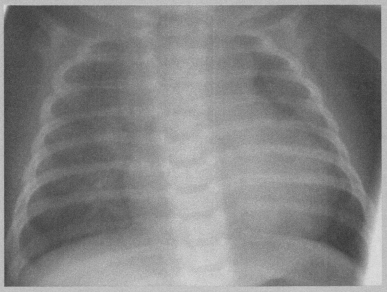

For more information, see:

http://en.wikipedia.org/wiki/Ventricular_septal_defect

http://www.nlm.nih.gov/medlineplus/ency/article/001099.htm

For your notes and thoughts

Clinical examination station: case 5

Cystic fibrosis

Information given to the candidate

You enter the station and the examiner introduces you to Joanna, a 12-year-old girl. She is sitting on a couch with her mother by her side.

Your task

You are asked to examine her respiratory system.

You are allowed to talk to the patient but are not allowed to ask any history unless allowed by the examiner.

You have nine minutes to complete the station; a warning bell will be given at seven minutes.

The examination

You introduce yourself to Joanna and her mother, explain to them what you will be doing and obtain a verbal consent to perform the examination.

You explain that hand hygiene has been adhered to, or alternatively use alcohol gel in front of child and parent.

Explain to Joanna that you will ask for her help in simple language.

On general inspection

- There are medications on the side table, Creon (pancreatic enzymes), and some antibiotics. There is a peak flow meter.
- Growth chart with height and weight plotted – on 50th centile.
- A long line is seen on the right chest wall.
- Joanna's height and weight are appropriate.

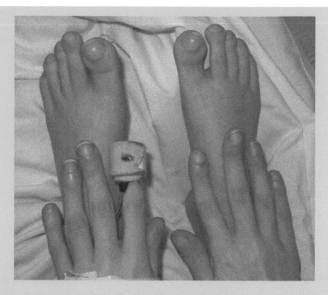

General physical and systemic examination

- Gross clubbing.
- No cyanosis.
- Chest wall symmetrical.
- Equal air entry; no additional sounds.
- Heart sounds normal, no murmur.
- Abdomen is soft; liver and spleen not palpable.

Confirm that the medicines and the growth chart on the side table are Joanna's.

You turn to the examiner and summarise your findings.

Following this you should be prepared for further discussion with the examiner.

Findings

You have examined Joanna, a 12-year-old girl. She looks well. On general inspection you note there are some medications on the side table, including Creon. Her height and weight are on the 50th centile. Joanna is comfortable at rest and has a long line visible on the right chest wall. There is gross clubbing, but no cyanosis. Chest shape is normal with normal air entry and no additional sounds. The rest of the examination is normal with no heapto-spleenomegaly.

You do not need to stop and can move on to your impression.

In your opinion Joanna has cystic fibrosis. She is on regular medication and is very well controlled, evident from her appropriate growth. You would like to check her peak flow.

What is expected from the candidate

The candidate should:

- introduce themself to Joanna and her mother
- request verbal consent to perform the examination
- perform hand hygiene procedures
- keep the patient at ease and give simple and easy to understand commands
- inspect and comment on observations
- work through and conclude differential pathologies
- be able to correlate the findings and discuss aetiology and management.

Further information

Cystic fibrosis

- There are about 8,000 patients with cystic fibrosis in the UK.
- Autosomal recessive – 1:4 chance of each child of 'carrier' parents being affected. 1:4 applies to each pregnancy.
- Median survival of babies born today with CF is 40 years.

Diagnosis

- Gold standard is sweat test with sweat chloride > 60 mmol.
- Faecal elastase in presence of pancreatic insufficiency. 15% of CF patients are pancreatic sufficient.
- DNA analysis.
- Neonatal screening – checks for immune-reactive trypsin (IRT).

Management

GPs have a central role, though overall care is provided by multidisciplinary teams consisting of specialist doctors, nurses, dieticians, physiotherapists and psychologists. Children are seen regularly with yearly evaluation of bloods, lung function and metabolic profile. Other treatments include:

- Respiratory therapies:
  - Chest physiotherapy. Family members are taught how to perform.
  - Mucoactive agents are used to clear secretions eg. dornase alpha, hypertonic saline.
  - Antibiotics – given orally, intravenously or nebulised. Prophylaxis is to reduce incidence of colonisation by staphylococci and pseudomonas aeruginosa.
  - Oxygen supplementation at home

- Gastrointestinal management:
  - High-calorie diet. Nasogastric feeding or a gastrostomy for adequate intake of calories are necessary for some patients.
  - Pancreatic enzymes are given as required.
  - Vitamin supplements are given, especially fat-soluble: A, D, E, K.
  - Constipation is treated with appropriate laxative treatment.
- Other complications:
  - Bone problems – osteoporosis.
  - Liver
  - Diabetes develops in the second decade and is managed by insulin and dietary restrictions.
- New therapies:
  - New mucoactive agents
  - Therapies targeting basic effects of CFTR protein function.

For more information, see:

http://www.nhs.uk/Conditions/cystic-fibrosis/Pages/Introduction.aspx

http://en.wikipedia.org/wiki/Cystic_fibrosis

For your notes and thoughts

Clinical examination station: case 6

Exacerbation of asthma

Information given to the candidate

You enter the examination room and the examiner introduces you to David, an eight-year-old boy. David is sitting on a chair wearing shorts but the upper half of his body is unclothed. He looks comfortable and there is a spacer and metered dose inhaler device lying on the table.

The examiner explains that David's father is worried about his worsening breathing and frequent coughs for the past two months.

Your task

You must examine David's respiratory system.

You are allowed to talk to the patient but not allowed to ask any questions about his condition.

You have nine minutes to complete the station; a warning bell will be given at seven minutes.

(**Note:** patients who are stable and recovering from an acute illness such as exacerbation of asthma, pneumonia etc. may come for exam from an inpatient ward.)

Examination

You introduce yourself to David and his father, explain to them what you will be doing and obtain a verbal consent to conduct an examination.

You explain that hand hygiene has been adhered to, or alternatively use alcohol gel in front of child and parent.

You explain to David that you will ask for his help in simple language.

General physical examination

- You look around the room and notice an MDI and spacer on the table. There is also a peak flow meter. He has name bands attached on both his wrists and you realise that he is an inpatient.

- He appears mildly tachypneic. Respiratory rate is 28/min.

- Pulse rate 104/min.
- No clubbing.
- No pallor or cyanosis (tip of tongue).
- No recessions or scars but minimal tracheal tug.
- Antero-posterior diameter of the chest wall not increased.
- Apex beat is on the left 5th inter-costal space.
- Expansion is limited but equal and symmetrical at the front and back.

You then explain to David that you would like to tap his chest like a drum and proceed to percuss the chest, but the examiner asks you to auscultate only and you note a scattered wheeze, bilateral ronchii and an increase in the duration of the expiratory phase on the back.

You turn to the examiner and summarise your findings.

Following this you should be prepared for further discussion with the examiner.

Findings

You have examined David, an eight-year-old boy. He is mildly tachypneic, not cyanosed, and has no clubbing. His chest is symmetrical and seems hyper-inflated ie. as if in inspiration. He has a scattered wheeze and ronchii on both sides. There is a spacer and an MDI on the side table. In your opinion David is likely to be recovering from an acute exacerbation of asthma and is probably an inpatient in the ward, as suggested by the name bands on his wrists.

What is expected from the candidate

The candidate should:

- introduce themself to David and his father and request verbal consent to perform an examination
- perform hand hygiene procedures
- note medical devices present near the patient
- enquire whether David is well and mention the inpatient wrist band
- keep the patient at ease and give simple and easy to understand commands
- count respiratory rate for a full 30 seconds with a watch when requested
- examine patient on the couch
- kneel or sit down by the side of the couch, and they should not stoop over the patient
- comment about the apex beat, chest expansion, respiratory distress and findings on auscultation.

Further information

Asthma is a common disease in childhood. Know it well. It makes a significant part of work in general practice.

You should know the current British Thoracic Society's and SIGN guidelines on diagnosis and management.

You can assess the severity of a child's asthma quickly by asking:

- How the child is doing at school – how many days have they missed?
- Can he run as fast as his friends? If there was a race in your class where would he come?
- Can he keep pace with his peers in PE and games or does he need to stop earlier?
- What games does he play? (If he says football, try to find what position he plays (eg. goalkeeper) to determine the activity level).
- Does he cough at night and does he wake in the night with a cough?

What investigation can be useful in an acute attack?

- Saturation monitoring.
- PEFR (peak expiratory flow rate) pre and post-bronchodilator therapy.
- CXR to rule an infective cause for the exacerbation.

Long-term management should include:

- Monitoring, preferably with a paediatrician and an asthma nurse specialist or GP with special interest.
- A steroid inhaler (preventer).
- Checking inhaler technique.
- Growth monitoring: height and weight.

The PEFR can be performed by a child older than five years of age on simple explanation and correct demonstration of the technique. As a rough guide, for a height of 110cm, expected PEFR will be 150, and then for every 10cm increase in height the PEFR should increase by 50mm. So, for a 120cm tall child, PEFR is 200; 130cm tall child it is 250 and so on (Source APLS manual, 4th edition).

Check the British Thoracic Society's guidelines to find out about stepping up and down treatment for a child with asthma.

For more information, see:

http://www.brit-thoracic.org.uk/guidelines-and-quality-standards/asthma-guideline/

For your notes and thoughts

Clinical examination station: case 7

Spina bifida

Information given to the candidate

You enter the examination station and the examiner introduces you to six-month-old Grace and her parents. Grace has been unsettled during the night and has come for an appointment. She is lying on the couch.

Your task

Conduct a general physical examination and any relevant system examination.

You are allowed to talk to the patient but are not allowed to ask any history unless allowed by the examiner.

You have nine minutes to complete the station; a warning bell will be given at seven minutes.

The examination

You introduce yourself to Grace and her parents. Explain to them what you will be doing and obtain verbal consent to perform the examination.

You explain that hand hygiene has been adhered to, or alternatively use alcohol gel in front of child and parent.

On general inspection Grace looks well, pink, and is not distressed. She is smiling at her mother.

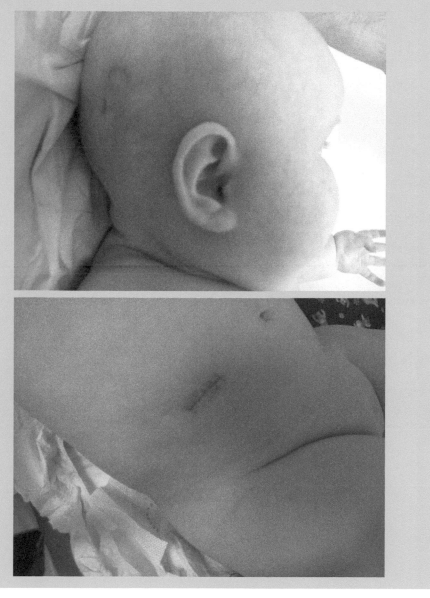

General physical and systemic examination

- Grace is alert and responds to your speech and facial gestures.
- Her abdomen is moving with respiration.
- There is a scar in the right lumbar region – one inch long.
- Her chest is clear with normal heart sounds.
- Anterior fontanelle is flat, not tense, and you can feel pulsation.
- Feeling round her skull, you note a swelling behind her right ear and on further inspection:
  - there is a curved scar, three centimetres long
  - you notice a soft swelling, 1.5cm across, which compresses.

You ask her parents' permission to examine her back and they agree:

- You note a surgical scar in the lower lumbar region – upper sacral area.
- Grace retracts her legs on tickling her soles.

You ask for a patellar hammer – the examiner asks you why and then tells you not to use the hammer.

You ask to look into her ears – examiner asks you why and then tells you tympanic membranes are normal.

On completing your examination you take a few seconds to collect your thoughts and then turn to the examiner to summarise your findings.

Findings

You have examined Grace who is six months old. She is alert and seems comfortable at present. She has scars on her scalp, a scar on the abdomen and a healing scar on the back. Her fontanelle is not full or tense. Her chest is clear and her heart sounds are normal.

You do not need to stop and can move on to your impression.

In your opinion she has spina bifida with a ventriculo-peritoneal shunt. There is no obvious cause for her being unsettled during the night.

Following this you should be prepared for discussion as the case is simple and you should have ample time left till the bell rings.

What is expected from the candidate

The candidate should:

- acknowledge Grace and introduce themself to Grace's parents
- request verbal consent
- make it known that hand hygiene has been carried out before touching the patient
- follow a logical sequence to the examination
- keep the patient at ease
- inspect and comment on observations
- reach a diagnosis of spina bifida
- work through and evaluate different pathologies
- be able to correlate their findings and discuss aetiology and management.

Further information

Spina bifida describes a variety of congenital defects in the spinal column of a foetus.

Myelomeningocele

The spinal column remains open along the vertebral bodies. The membranes and spinal cord push out to create a sac. Myelomeningocele can undergo surgical repair. The nervous system is usually damaged resulting in a range of symptoms:

- Partial or total paralysis of the lower limbs.
- Bowel and urinary incontinence.
- Loss of skin sensation.

Most babies with myelomeningocele develop hydrocephalus requiring a ventriculo – peritoneal shunt.

The child can be assisted with:

- physiotherapy and occupational therapy to improve day-to-day life and boost independence.
- technology, such as manual or electric wheelchairs
- computer software to help with schoolwork and writing.
- treatments for bowel and urinary problems.

Spina bifida occulta

No obvious sign of a malformation. There's a gap in one or more vertebrae, but the skin is intact. The nerves and spinal cord are normal and the child may experience mild or no symptoms.

Spina bifida occulta in children is not detected until an x-ray is performed, often for an unrelated condition.

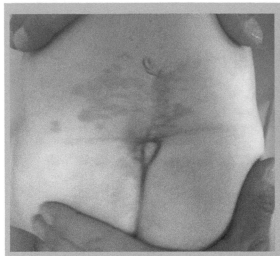

Repaired meningomyelocele

CT Scan showing dialated ventricles, keeping with hydrocephalus

The cause of spina bifida and other open neural tube defects (OPND) is unknown, however, mothers taking enough folic acid at the time of conception and during pregnancy can reduce the risk. Folic acid is now a mandatory vitamin additive in cereals and some food grains eg. breakfast cereals.

For more information, see:

http://www.nhs.uk/Conditions/Spina-bifida/Pages/Introduction.aspx

http://www.nhs.uk/Conditions/Hydrocephalus/Pages/Treatment.aspx

http://www.childrenshospital.org/az/Site1062/mainpageS1062P1.html

For your notes and thoughts

Clinical examination station: case 8

Facial palsy

Information given to the candidate

On entering the station you are introduced to Tony. He is eight years old and he has come with his mother due to difficulties with speech and drooling of saliva for the past two days.

Your task

Conduct a general physical examination and any other relevant system examination.

You are allowed to talk to the patient but are not allowed to ask any history unless allowed by the examiner.

You have nine minutes to complete the station; a warning bell will be given at seven minutes.

The examination

You introduce yourself, explain to Tony and his mother what you will be doing and obtain a verbal consent to perform the examination.

You explain that hand hygiene has been adhered to, or alternatively use alcohol gel in front of child and parent.

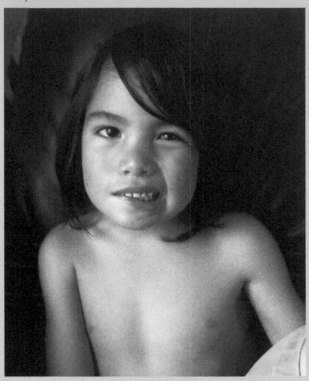

On general inspection

- Tony looks comfortable.
- His growth seems to be age appropriate but you would like to plot him on a growth chart.

General physical and systemic examination

- There is an obvious facial asymmetry. Right-sided naso-labial fold is less prominent.
- You assess the motor component of the facial (VII) cranial nerve – raise eyebrows, strength of eye lid closure, blow out cheeks and smile showing the teeth.
- Tony is unable to close his right eye properly.

- The angle of his mouth on the left side is deviated when compared to the right side.
- There are no vesicles around the ear – herpes zoster (Ramsay Hunt syndrome).
- You can find no features of mumps or otitis media.
- You offer to measure blood pressure.
- There is no circular erythematous rash with a bite mark (erythema migrans – Lyme disease).
- You ask Tony or his mother about:
  - any hyperacusis
  - decreased tearing
  - taste disturbances
  - history of travel to a farm or a forest recently (tick bite).

You conclude your examination, take a few seconds to gather your thoughts and turn to the examiner to summarise your findings.

Findings

You have examined eight-year-old Tony who has right-sided facial palsy. He is normotensive. There are no features suggestive of mumps, lyme disease or Ramsay Hunt syndrome.

You can move on to your impression.

Your findings are consistent with right-sided lower motor neurone facial nerve palsy, possibly secondary to Bell's palsy.

Following this you should be prepared for discussion as the case is simple and you should have ample time left till the bell rings.

What is expected from the candidate

The candidate should:

- introduce themself to Tony and his mother
- request verbal consent to perform the examination
- make it known that hand hygiene procedures have been carried before touching the patient
- follow a logical sequence to the examination
- keep the patient at ease and give simple commands
- work through and evaluate different pathologies
- try to elicit features supporting/excluding possible aetiologies of facial nerve palsy
- be able to correlate their findings and discuss aetiology and management.

Further reading

There are many causal factors associated with facial palsy:

- Birth – forceps delivery.
- Moebius syndrome (upper motor neurone lesion).
- Idiopathic – Bell's palsy, autoimmunity.
- Infections – mumps, otitis media, lyme disease, Ramsay Hunt syndrome (herpes zoster).
- Trauma – basal skull fracture, facial trauma.
- Metabolic – hyperthyroidism, hypertension.
- Tumours – leukaemia, cholesteatoma.
- Others – Guillain Barre syndrome (usually bilateral), cerebral palsy (usually upper motor neurone lesion).

In upper motor neurone (UMN) facial palsy the forehead is spared due to bilateral nerve innervations.

Total facial palsy is demonstrated in lower motor neurone palsy (LMN).

In unilateral lesion the angle of the mouth classically deviates to the normal side.

Treatment of Bell's palsy is controversial. The prognosis is fair, with complete recovery in about 80% of the cases, 15% experience some kind of permanent nerve damage and five per cent remain with severe long-term effects. Possible treatments include:

- eye protection – eye pads, artificial tears, eye drops
- prednisolone – 10–14 days
- physiotherapy for some cases.

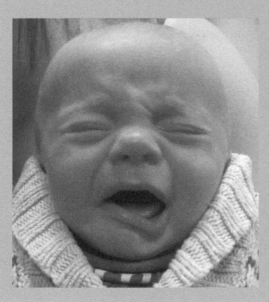

Ramsay Hunt syndrome

Ramsay Hunt syndrome is a complication of shingles. It is estimated to affect five in 100,000 people every year.

Lyme disease

Lyme disease is a bacterial infection that is spread to humans by infected ticks. The earliest and most common symptom is a pink or red circular rash that develops around the area of the bite, three to 30 days after someone is bitten. The rash is often described as looking like a bull's-eye on a dart board.

For more information, see:

http://www.ncbi.nlm.nih.gov/pmc/articles/PMC2440925/

http://www.nhs.uk/Conditions/Shingles/Pages/Complications.aspx

http://www.nhs.uk/conditions/Lyme-disease/Pages/Introduction.aspx

For your notes and thoughts

Clinical examination station: case 9

Neurofibromatosis

Information given to the candidate

On entering the station you are introduced to Nicola, nine years old. She has come with her mother for a routine review.

Your task

Conduct a general physical examination and any other relevant system examination.

You are allowed to talk to the patient but are not allowed to ask any history unless allowed by the examiner.

You have nine minutes to complete the station; a warning bell will be given at seven minutes.

The examination

You introduce yourself to Nicola and her mother, explain what you will be doing and obtain a verbal consent.

Explain that hand hygiene has been adhered to, or alternatively use alcohol gel in front of child and parent.

On general inspection:

- ■ Nicola looks comfortable.
- ■ Her growth seems to be age appropriate but you would like to plot her on a growth chart.

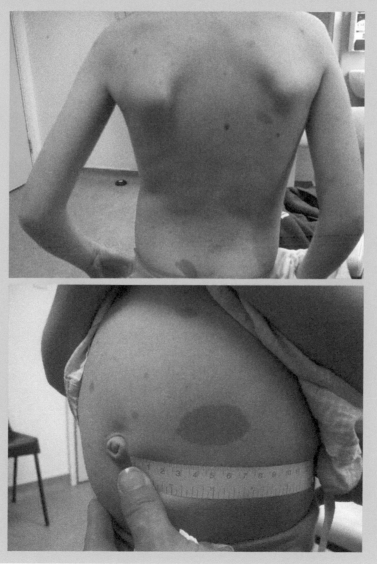

General physical and systemic examination

- There are brown-pigmented patches of different sizes distributed all over the body. You would like to measure the sizes of these skin lesions.
- There are eight lesions that are more than 5mm in size.
- Axillary freckles are seen.
- No neurofibromas or plexiform neurofibromas seen.
- No obvious bone lesions.
- You can find no evidence of precocious puberty.
- Measure her blood pressure (association with renal artery stenosis and phaeochromocytoma).
- You refer her to the ophthalmology team in a view of possible Lisch nodules in the iris.
- You ask her mother if she has:
    - any first-degree relative with a similar condition.
    - had a brain scan (MRI) and regular hearing assessment.
    - any genetic counselling.

You conclude your examination and turn to the examiner to summarise your findings.

Findings

You have examined nine-year-old Nicola who seems to be an appropriate size for her age. She has eight café-au-lait patches that are more than 5mm in size. She also has axillary freckles but no obvious bony deformities or neurofibromas. She does not show any evidence of precocious puberty and her father suffers from a similar condition.

You can move on to your impression.

Your findings are consistent with Neurofibromatosis type I.

Following this, you should be prepared for discussion as the case is simple and you should have ample time left till the bell rings.

What is expected from the candidate

The candidate should:
- introduce themself to Nicola and her mother
- request verbal consent to conduct the examination
- make it known that hand hygiene procedures have been carried out before touching the patient
- follow a logical sequence to the examination
- keep the patient at ease and give simple commands
- objectively look for some of the many associations of neurofibromatosis
- display knowledge about the diagnostic criteria
- be able to correlate the findings and discuss aetiology and management.

Further information

Neurofibromatosis (Von Recklinghausen disease/NF) is an autosomal dominant inherited condition, however 50% are new mutations. The gene is located on chromosome 17q.

NF1 constitutes the majority of cases (90%). The severity can vary from mild with no serious health problems, to significant systemic manifestations of a severe form.

Diagnosis

Two or more of the following seven criteria are required:
1. Six or more café-au-lait patches (prepubertal size >5mm but post pubertal >15mm).
2. Axillary freckles.
3. Two or more neurofibromas or one plexiform neurofibroma.
4. Two or more lisch nodules in iris.
5. Bone lesion.
6. Sphenoid dysplasia.
7. Bowing of the tibia.
8. Optic glioma.
9. First-degree relative with NF1.

In the normal population, one or two café-au-lait spot patches may be seen.

Subcutaneous neurofibromas may be tender.

The following may be associated with NF1:

- Tumours – Wilm's tumour, leukaemia, phaeochromocytoma.
- CVS – hypertension, pulmonary stenosis, cardiomyopathy.
- Renal artery stenosis.
- CNS – epilepsy.
- Macrocephaly.
- Attention deficit hyperactivity disorder (ADHD).
- Precocious puberty.

Management

Management depends upon the extent and the site of the clinical involvement.

Children with mild NF1, can feel self-conscious about their appearance leading to stress and possible depression.

Several organisations and support groups offer helplines, online forums and blogs written by people with the condition.

These organisations include The Neuro Foundation and the Children's Tumor Foundation.

For more information, see http://www.nhs.uk/Conditions/Neurofibromatosis/Pages/Symptoms.aspx

For your notes and thoughts

Clinical examination station: case 10

Tuberous sclerosis

Information given to the candidate

Nine-year-old Oliver presented with resistant epilepsy needing multiple anti-epileptic medications, and he also has significant learning difficulties. He has been brought to the surgery by his mother.

Your task

Conduct a general physical examination and any other relevant system examination to reach a diagnosis or differential diagnoses.

You are allowed to talk to the patient but are not allowed to ask any history unless given permission by the examiner.

You have nine minutes to complete the station; a warning bell will be given at seven minutes.

The examination

Introduce yourself, explain what you will be doing and obtain a verbal consent.

You explain that hand hygiene has been adhered to, or alternatively use alcohol gel in front of child and parent.

On general inspection:

- Oliver looks well.
- His growth seems to be age appropriate but you would like to plot him on a growth chart.
- He does not seem to be interacting with the environment appropriately.

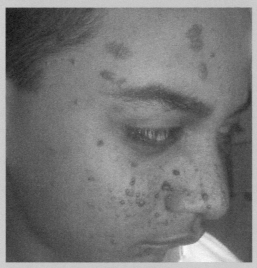

General physical and systemic examination

- Multiple erythematous papular nodular lesions are seen over the face.
- Some of them have irregular margins (adenoma sebaceum).
- Multiple depigmented macules of varying sizes are seen mainly on the trunk (ash leaf macule).
- Mid-line sternotomy scar.
- Irregular thickened area with leathery texture over the lower lumbar area (shagreen patch).

You perform a basic developmental assessment – speech, co-ordination skills.

Ater asking the examiner's permission you ask Oliver's mother:

- whether Oliver had a cardiac surgery to remove a heart tumour
- if he attends a school with special needs
- if he has had MRI (brain) and renal scans.

You turn to the examiner and summarise your findings.

Findings

You have examined nine-year-old Oliver who looks comfortable. He has adenoma sebaceum, ash leaf macules and a shagreen patch. Oliver also has a sternotomy scar and developmental delay.

Your findings are consistent with tuberous sclerosis and the sternotomy scar may be for removal of a rhabdomyoma.

What is expected from the candidate

The candidate should:

- introduce themself to Oliver and his mother
- request verbal consent to perform the examination
- make it known that hand hygiene procedures have been carried out before touching the patient
- follow a logical sequence to the examination
- keep the patient at ease and give simple commands
- objectively look for classical skin lesions
- be familiar with the condition, but they are not expected to know all the minor details
- be able to discuss briefly how to manage a child with chronic disability.

Further information

Tuberous sclerosis is a rare genetic condition with autosomal dominant inheritance. 80% are due to new mutations.

Benign tumours develop in different parts of the body and can be seen in:

- the skin
- the brain
- the heart
- the eyes
- the kidneys
- the lungs.

Diagnosis

Diagnosis is clinical and requires two major criteria, or one major with two minor features. Major features are in italics.

- Skin manifestations:
  - *Adenoma sebaceum.* (Usually after three years of age.)
  - *Ash leaf macules.*
  - *Shagreen patches.*
  - *Ungualm/periungual fibromas.*
  - Localised patch of white hair.
- CVS – *rhabdomyomas.*
- CNS – epilepsy, development delay, *gliomas.*
- Renal – *angiomyolipomas,* polycystic kidney disease.
- Lung – *lymphangioleiomyomatosis* (LAM).
- Retina – phakoma.
- Behavioural – ADHD, autism.

Investigations

- MRI (brain) for cortical tubers and other CNS lesions.
- EEG.
- Renal USS.
- Echocardiography, ECG.
- Fundoscopy.

Management

- Multidisciplinary.
- Anti-epileptics.
- Behaviour management.
- Special schooling.

A key worker (health visitor and social worker) will be the point of contact with the various support services available.

For more information, see:

http://www.nhs.uk/conditions/Tuberous-sclerosis/Pages/Introduction.aspx

http://www.nhs.uk/Conditions/Tuberous-sclerosis/Pages/Treatment.aspx

For your notes and thoughts

Focused history and management station

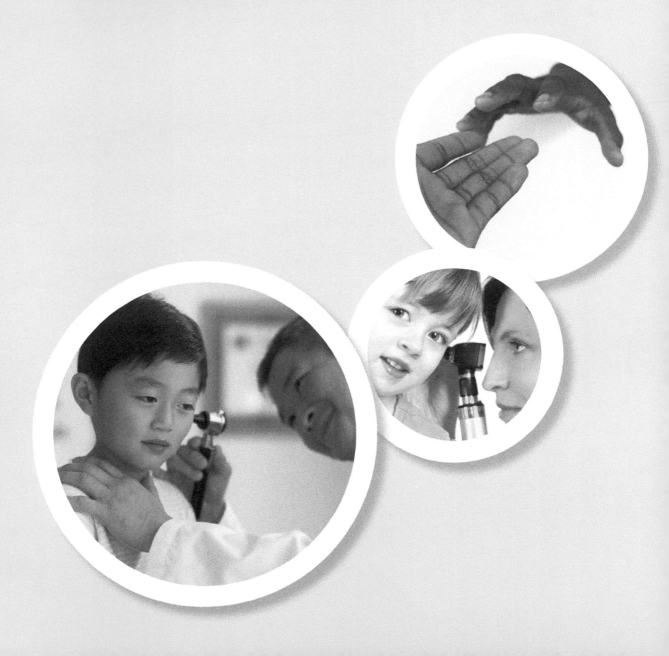

Focused history and management station

This section should be conducted with a role-player, who will usually take on the role of one of the patient's parents.

The candidate should read the information in the first box, but not in the second so that they do not know what to expect from the role-player.

They should investigate the role-player to extract as much information as they can. The role-player, meanwhile, will also have access to the information in the third box so they can 'mark' how well the candidate performs.

This is a nine-minute station. You will have six minutes with the patient (a warning bell will be given at five minutes). The examiner will observe you during this time.

You will then have three minutes with the examiner for discussion.

Focused history and management station: case 1

Enuresis

Information given to the candidate

You are a GP registrar and Jonny is a six-year-old boy. His mother has come to speak to you as Jonny has started bedwetting recently, having had been previously dry for three months. His physical examination is normal. He is growing well along 50th centile. His blood sugar is 5.2mmol/L. Urine dipstix is 'normal' with no sugar or blood.

Your task

You must take a focused history and give a reasonable management plan to Jonny's mother.

This is a nine-minute station. You will have six minutes with the patient (a warning bell will be given at five minutes). The examiner will observe you during this time. You will then have three minutes with the examiner for discussion.

Information available to the role-player

You are Ms Jones, Jonny's mother:

- Jonny was dry for three months but has started bedwetting again.
- He has moved to a different school recently.
- He opens his bowels every fourth day (and if shown a stool chart you recognise Jonny's stool as type 2).
- Jonny's dad was dry at night by nine years of age.
- He is doing well at school and is not being bullied. He remains extremely active and plays football two days a week.
- You are worried that he may be diabetic and need reassurance about this.
- Jonny may be offered an ultrasound scan, however you need an explanation that this is familial delay in getting bladder control.

What is expected from the candidate

The candidate should:

- introduce themself to the examiner
- have a fluent and structured approach
- explore Ms Jones' concerns regarding Jonny's bedwetting
- ask the about '4T' symptoms for diabetes:
  - thirst
  - thinner
  - tiredness
  - (increased) toileting
- reassure Ms Jones that this is not diabetes following a normal blood sugar result, and the candidate should not waste too much time gathering history about diabetes
- ask about any history of constipation and address this while giving a management plan to Jonny's mother (or later discuss this with the examiner)
- explore psychological issues such as bullying or family difficulties etc.
- ask about family history of late bladder control
- explain enuresis (late bladder control) in Jonny and the candidate may ask for a renal ultrasound scan
- offer to refer Jonny to a continence nurse specialist and initiate laxative therapy
- offer appropriate follow-up plan.

Further information

Enuresis is a common presentation for clinicians looking after children, and it often presents in children from families with a history of the condition.

The following terms are commonly used:

- Nocturnal enuresis: a child five years and above suffers incontinence while asleep.
- Primary nocturnal enuresis: a child who has previously been dry for less than six months.
- Secondary nocturnal enuresis: a child who has previously been dry for at least six months.

The management of enuresis is based on:

- Checking family dynamics and history of enuresis in parents and siblings.
- Checking sleeping arrangements at home, such as sleeping in bunk beds.
- Addressing constipation.
- Bladder training by establishing a regular pattern.
- Intervention aimed at enuresis:
  - Alarms.
  - Medication – desmopressin.

It is suggested that candidates read the NICE clinical guidelines 111 (2010) entitled *Nocturnal enuresis: the management of bedwetting in children and young people.*

For more information, see:

http://www.nice.org.uk/cg111

http://www.eric.org.uk/Training/nocturnal_enuresis

For your notes and thoughts

Focused history and management station: case 2

Migraine

Information given to the candidate

You are a GP registrar. Jamie is a six-year-old boy whose mother has come to speak to you regarding his headaches. Jamie is at school today but was examined by your colleague yesterday afternoon and had a completely normal neurological examination. Please take a focused history and give a reasonable management plan to Jamie's mother.

This is a nine-minute station. You will have six minutes with the patient (a warning bell will be given at five minutes). The examiner will observe you during this time. You will then have three minutes with the examiner for discussion.

Information available to the role-player

You are Ms Smith, Jamie's mother.

- Jamie suffers from headaches every other week, especially in the afternoon.
- He never wakes up with a headache first thing in the morning and he does not wake up during the night with headaches.
- He sometimes feels nauseous before the headache and needs to sleep in a dark room.
- Paracetamol helps the headache but you are reluctant to give it every day.
- You, your sisters and your parents suffer from migraines.
- Your friend's child has recently been diagnosed with a brain tumour and you are worried about it.
- You need to be reassured that it is not something serious such as brain tumour.
- You can ask for a CT scan, but do not need to push for it.

What is expected from the candidate

The candidate should:

- introduce themself to the examiner
- have a fluent and structured approach
- explore Ms Smith's concerns regarding Jamie's headaches
- ask about red flag symptoms (eg. waking up with headaches, vomiting, disturbance in vision, deterioration in behaviour etc)
- explore family history of headaches, especially migraine
- explain migraine in clear and simple language
- not agree to act scan but adequately reassure Ms Smith that Jamie's symptoms are not due to brain tumours
- offer appropriate prophylaxis and make a follow-up plan.

Further information

Headaches are common in children and are generally benign.

The red flag symptoms to be aware of are:

- vomiting (persistent/recurrent)
- waking up with headache in the morning
- gait disturbances
- deterioration in behaviour
- deterioration in school performance or handwriting.

'HeadSmart' give symptoms and signs that should be looked for in children where there is a concern of possible brain tumour.

Candidates should specifically ask about family history of migraines and the timing and pattern of headaches in the child. There is a 30% chance of a child being a sufferer if one parent experiences migraine, and a 60% chance if both parents do.

Migraines are common in children, with some studies suggesting one in 10 children suffer from them. There can be history of:

- nausea and vomiting – with possible diagnosis of 'cyclical vomiting'
- abdominal pain
- dizziness
- aura, visual disturbance, sensitivity to light
- excessive tiredness.

Triggers

- Irregular eating, leading to dehydration.
- Anxiety and stress.
- Certain foods, such as chocolates, caffeine and citrus fruits.
- Watching too much television.
- Puberty in girls.

Keeping a symptom diary is very useful in diagnosis and treatment. Treatment is based on life-style adjustments and drugs, including:

- Analgesics – paracetamol, ibuprofen.
- Pizotifen.
- Sumatraptan.

For more information, see:

http://www.nhs.uk/Livewell/headaches/Pages/Headachesinchildren.aspx

http://www.mayoclinic.com/health/headaches-in-children/DS01132

http://www.headsmart.org.uk/admin/uploads/Headsmart-Symptom-card-final.pdf

http://www.nhs.uk/ipgmedia/national/migraine%20action/assets/migraineinchildrenandyoungpeople.pdf

For your notes and thoughts

Focused history and management station: case 3

Behaviour problems

Information given to the candidate

You are a GP and you are talking to Miss Harwood, Ollie's mother. Ollie is five years old. Ollie's mother is worried that her son is extremely hyperactive and difficult to manage at home.

Your task

Take a focused history and discuss your management plan with the examiner.

You are not expected to examine the patient or discuss management. You may answer any queries that may arise during the discussion.

This is a nine-minute station. You will have six minutes with the patient (a warning bell will be given at five minutes). The examiner will observe you during this time. You will then have three minutes with the examiner for discussion.

Information available to role-player

- Ollie is always 'on the go' and does not stop throughout the day. According to his mother he does not listen or obey commands given by her.
- As Ollie has no sense of danger, Miss Harwood finds it difficult to take him to public places and supermarkets.
- She usually gives one-to-one supervision all the time.
- He cannot sit in one place or complete a given task.
- He likes playing with his games console and likes to build Lego structures, and when engaged in these activities he is able to concentrate for long periods.
- His past medical history is unremarkable and he is not on any long-term medication.
- His birth history was unremarkable.
- His development is normal and he is fully immunised.

- He is independent with self-help skills. Although he usually goes to bed late, he sleeps through the night.
- Apart from normal sibling rivalry, Ollie likes his sister.
- Miss Harwood is a single mother and has a younger daughter who is three years old. She is unemployed and receives benefits. Ollie's father is not allowed to visit the family due to previous domestic violence. The family has a named social worker. She is upset about Ollie's behaviour and unable to cope with the situation.
- His school and class teacher have no major concerns. He has lot of friends in the school and is very social. His learning is average, but he is particularly good at maths. He usually respects adults.

What is expected from the candidate

The candidate should:

- introduce themself to the examiner and the patient
- address Ollie and his mother by their names
- explore Miss Harwood's main concerns
- explore the support she receives
- obtain details about Ollie's activities and his daily routine at home
- ask about his birth history and development milestones to rule out any possible underlying neurological condition
- gather details about family history and social history
- gather details about schooling and any concerns
- not repeat the entire history (do not waste your time – you were being observed) summarise the problems identified and supporting facts
- discuss Miss Harwood's main concerns
- discuss the plan of management:
    - Observe the child during the consultation to get an idea of his behaviour – usually ADHD children are difficult to keep in the room.
    - Perform neurological and systemic examinations to exclude any underlying pathology.
    - Request a school report (this allows you to get an accurate idea about him in the school).
    - Recognise that the problems are mainly observed at home.
    - Explain the need for a structured approach at home.
    - Increase outdoor activities for him (suggest activities).
    - Access a local family centre for parenting courses on how to manage difficult children at home.
    - Arrange a common assessment framework (CAF).
    - Liaise with the health visitor and the social worker.

Further information

Attention deficit hyperactivity disorders (ADHD) affect two to five per cent of school children in UK, and is more common in boys. It is being increasingly recognised and diagnosed.

Common symptom include:

- inattentiveness
- impulsiveness
- hyperactivity
- a short attention span and being easily distracted
- restlessness/constant fidgeting.

Diagnosis is usually between three and seven years of age.

The following are considered when assessing children for ADHD:

- Hyperactivity – most children with ADHD cannot sit still, they fidget, run around or move excessively.

- Inattention – a child does not finish things once started and does not engage with a play activity for long.

- Impulsivity – a child acts without thinking of consequences. One-to-one supervision is required and they struggle to function in group situations.

These symptoms should persist for more than six months in more than one setting eg. school, home.

Management

- Connor's questionnaire – a process of interviews, observations and assessments. There are three Connor's rating scales: one is designed for parents, another for teachers, and one asks adolescents to rate their own behaviour. The final results are compiled in an easy-to-interpret graph.

- Behaviour and family therapy.

- Dietary modifications – food colourings, dairy products, sugar, chocolate and fried food should be avoided.

- In severe cases:

  - Drug therapy/stimulants eg. methylphenidate (Ritalin).
  - School with special needs for severe cases.

For more information, see:

http://www.nhs.uk/Conditions/Attention-deficit-hyperactivity-disorder/Pages/Introduction.aspx

http://www.nice.org.uk/cg72

For your notes and thoughts

Focused history and management station: case 4

Infantile colic

Information given to the candidate

You are a GP and you are talking to Emma, the mother of George, eight weeks old. Emma has come to see you without George as she feels he is not well, is not sleeping and is crying day and night.

Your task

Take a focused history and discuss your management plan with the examiner.

You are not expected to examine the patient. You should answer any queries that may arise during the discussion.

This is a nine-minute station. You will have six minutes with the patient; a warning bell will be given at five minutes. The examiner will observe you during this time. You will have three minutes with the examiner for discussion.

The examiner will focus on your understanding of disease management.

Information available to role-player

- Emma is 18 years old.
- George is Emma's first child.
- He was born by emergency caesarean section but stayed with Emma.
- Emma tried to breast feed but could not sustain it, and since the age of two weeks he has been on formula feed.
- He cries a lot and Emma therefore gives him many bottle feeds, sometimes more than 10 times a day.
- He vomits small amounts most of the time.
- His stools are hard and he opens his bowels once a day.
- He has dry skin.
- Emma has little support and her partner works at night and sleeps in the day time.
- She feels lonely and tired.
- She is very upset.

What is expected from the candidate

The candidate should:
- introduce themself to the parent and ask about George's well-being
- address George and Emma by their names
- explain and agree the agenda for the discussion
- get a dietary history of both George and Emma
- respond to Emma if she is crying/being upset
- not gather unnecessary history or information
- frequently summarise what is understood
- avoid monologues – they should encourage Emma to speak and not interfere frequently
- give a clear management plan and follow-up plans
- not use medical jargon
- not repeat the whole case history (do not waste your time – you were being observed)
- mention the working diagnosis with supporting facts
- consider postnatal depression instead of simply labelling her symptoms as tiredness and exhaustion
- reassure Emma that it is a temporary phase and that it will pass
- recommend that Emma try different teats, if she has not already done so, to alter flow rates
- mention contact and help from health visitor
- can use simethicone (Dentinox) but do not use dicycloverine (dicyclomine) (Merbentyl) due to potential respiratory difficulty and coma.

Further information

Infantile colic is common – around one in five babies, equally in both sexes, are affected.

It is more common before three months, lasts for three to four months, and usually resolves by six months.

There is no recognised cause. However:
- it is more common in bottle-fed babies
- avoiding dairy products gives relief
- hypoallergenic formula feeds can be a useful therapeutic measure
- family stress is associated with colic.

Lactose free milk is different and lactose intolerance is rare in babies with colic.

There is no test to confirm the diagnosis, hence it is a diagnosis of exclusion.

NICE guidelines advise urgent assessment of infants with colic to exclude causes such as Hirschsprung's disease or intestinal obstruction.

Medications are generally not recommended. Simethicone may be used, Merbentyl (dicycloverine) is to be avoided – NICE guidelines.

For more information, see:

http://www.pulse-learning.co.uk/clinical-modules/paediatrics/the-information-infant-colic-cpd-module

For your notes and thoughts

Focused history and management station: case 5

New onset diabetes

Information given to the candidate

You are a GP registrar. Jordan is nine years old. His mother is concerned that he is drinking too much water. His clothes have become loose and he has lost about 2kg in weight. Please take a focused history and explain your management plan to Jordan's mother.

This is a nine-minute station. You will have six minutes with the patient (a warning bell will be given at five minutes). The examiner will observe you during this time. You will then have three minutes with the examiner for discussion.

Information available to the role-player
- You are Mrs Hunt, Jordan's mother.
- Jordan has started bedwetting and drinking four litres of water/juice each day.
- Jordan's father has type 1 diabetes and you are worried that Jordan has now developed it.
- He is extremely tired and has lost weight.
- You are worried that Jordan is likely to have diabetes too.
- You need to be shown empathy and exhibit controlled emotions.

What is expected from the candidate

The candidate should:

- introduce themself to the examiner
- have a fluent and structured approach
- explore Mrs Hunt's concerns regarding Jordan's bedwetting and other symptoms
- ask about the 4T symptoms for diabetes: thirst, tiredness, thinner, increased toileting
- enquire about family history of diabetes
- explain about suspicion of new onset diabetes and refer to paediatric services immediately
- offer a blood sugar test but this should not delay referral
- offer support and appropriate follow-up plan
- empathise with Jordan's mother and ensure that she understands that Jordan will have the full support of the children's diabetes team at the hospital.

Further information

Diabetes is increasingly being diagnosed in children.

It is important that candidates are aware of the varied presentations of diabetes and have read the NICE guidelines 15 (2004), entitled *Type 1 Diabetes: Diagnosis and management of type 1 diabetes in children, young people and adults*. It is also important to remain aware of the 4Ts campaign by Diabetes UK.

Diabetes may also be used at the structured oral or communication stations.

For more information, see:

http://www.nhs.uk/Livewell/Diabetes/Pages/Diabetesandyourchild.aspx

http://www.nice.org.uk/cg15

http://www.diabetes.org.uk/

For your notes and thoughts

Child development station

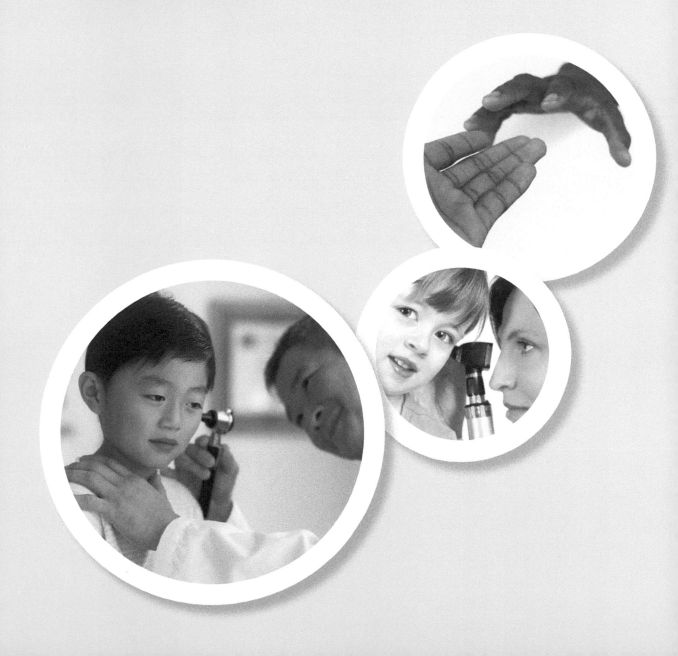

Child development station

Growth and development are two cornerstones of paediatric care. A child who is not developing or growing appropriately is of as much concern as any other clinical disease process in the body. Children are regularly monitored for their 'normal' growth and development until they reach adulthood and early identification is essential for improving the chances of remedial action, allowing an individual to reach their full potential.

The RCPCH gives special importance to development assessment and it is a mandatory station for the DCH examination. Candidates often view this station as the most difficult. A full and comprehensive development assessment, even by an experienced community paediatrician, can take a significant amount of time and the college therefore never expects candidates to complete one in a seven to nine-minute examination, as is often the case at other stations.

In the examination, candidates will therefore be asked to assess a particular aspect of development, demonstrate their skills and put in place an appropriate management plan for a child, normally below four years.

Candidates are therefore expected to be able to:

■ assess gross motor and fine motor skills

■ assess speech and language skills

■ anticipate and respond appropriately to age-related behaviour ie. separation anxiety etc.

■ estimate developmental age that is supported by the age-appropriate skills a child can demonstrate

■ identify those children who may not follow the normative stage

■ select the most appropriate tools for developmental assessment

■ note when a child is not able to perform a skill that might be expected of a slightly older child

■ discuss implications and appropriate management steps for a child with developmental concerns.

By the use of the development station, the RCPCH aims to assess a candidate's ability to perform developmental assessments by gathering information from various sources available, such as:

■ a clinical assessment of a child

■ a brief assessment of neurodisability if present

■ a supplementary history-taking from the parent, if appropriate

■ any other material provided in the station, such as:

    ■ parent-held records

    ■ growth charts

    ■ special equipment, wheel chair, braces, splints, hearing aids etc.

General instructions for the candidates (RCPCH guidelines):

1. The child will be below four years.

2. The examiner will decide the specific aspect of development to be assessed.

3. Toys and tools will be provided.

4. Psychometric testing need not be performed.

5. Six minutes will be provided to perform the examination and determine the nature and severity of any problem.

6. Candidates will be assessed by the degree of confidence they display during the examination.

7. Candidates should be able to outline a management plan.

8. Candidates should have a clear knowledge of the role of different members in a multidisciplinary team dealing with child developmental problems.

9. Candidates are expected to understand the principles of vision and hearing assessment.

Tips for candidates

The task will usually focus on one area of development. At the start of the station:

■ read/listen to the instructions carefully

■ make sure you clearly understand the task you are being asked to perform

■ **do not get confused** – if uncertain, clarify

■ it is not a history station, so do not ask too many questions

- you will be marked down for asking and not observing
- do not ask the age of the child unless it is mentioned in the task.

You should have a practised, slick and systematic approach to assessing development, as you should at all clinical stations. It should never come across that you are doing a particular task for the first time:

- Improve your observation skills. You can show the examiner how efficient you are at picking up clues just by 'observing' a child.
- Describe, in your mind, any child that you see for practice. When preparing for my exam, I used to describe any child I came across in a set format I felt comfortable with. This simple but very useful tip will improve your fluency in describing a child in the examination situation.
- Observe the child as you enter the room, while you are greeting the examiner and the parent.
- Your first observations of the child can give you a lot of information ie. stranger anxiety, no eye contact, fixity with any object, walking, kicking a ball etc.
- Describe the child to the examiner as you go along (or until asked to stop/ clarify etc). This will keep both you and your examiner engaged.

It is important that you build a rapport, engage and work with the child:

- You will have to demonstrate your rapport with children by being able to engage them with objects to carry out specific activities.
- Choose simple objects like books, beads, blocks, balls, paper and crayons.
- Use **only one tool at a time** so as not to divert their attention.
- Remove it from sight when you wish to move on to next tool.
- Practise with these tools with any child you come across (at work or at home).
- Your instructions should be specific and simple to follow.
- You may ask the parent to give the instructions if the child is apprehensive or shy.
- Use simple commands and you may need to demonstrate the task, for example:
  - 'Let's play and draw a picture' – show what you expect.
  - 'Let's make a tower with these coloured blocks.'
  - 'Can you make a tower like me?'

- Do not be too fixed with one object. If the child does not like blocks, move on to something else. You can always come back later.
- **Do not lose the child's attention and do not let them get bored.**

There will be occasions when a child may be tired, fractious or just not ready to play ball. Don't panic. The examiner will usually allow you to ask some questions. If so:

- Work on **targeted questions** that you may be allowed to ask parents.
- Your questions should be clear and specific.
    - Do not ask **open questions** such as, 'what can your child do?'
    - Ask age-appropriate **closed questions**, such as:
        - can he climb stairs?
        - can she ride a tricycle?
        - can he drink from a cup?
        - can she hop?

By the end of the examination you should be able to give a balanced opinion on the task you were asked to perform, with supporting evidence that you have noted or that was demonstrated.

Timing and marking of this station:

- Total time for the station is nine minutes.
- Six minutes are spent with the child. The examiner will mark you for this section by observing your method, rapport, speed and professionalism.
- A time warning will be given at five minutes in order for you to conclude the examination.
- Three final minutes are used to discuss your findings and management plan with the examiner. Another set of marks is awarded here.

In the examination, the development station usually comes with one of three tasks.

The first task:

- To assess and grossly identify:
    - if a child's development is age appropriate or delayed
    - if there is any sign of neurodisability.

Quick tip: in fixing a developmental age, it might work better if you keep in mind what a child **cannot do** rather than what they **can** do. Below are some examples, but you can formulate your own parameters with tools you choose to use in the examination.

Example one:

- In gross motor assessment there may be developmental delay if Thomas:
    - cannot skip or hop: <five years
    - cannot ride a tricycle: <three years
    - cannot run freely: <two years
    - cannot walk steadily: <one year
    - cannot sit without support: <six months
    - cannot support head control : <three months

- In fine motor assessment using crayons, there may be developmental delay if Thomas:
    - cannot copy a _: <five years
    - cannot copy a _ : <four years
    - cannot copy a O : <three years
    - cannot copy a + : <two years
    - cannot imitate strokes: <one year

- With toy blocks, there may be developmental delay if Thomas:
    - cannot copy three-stair patterns with six blocks: <four to five years
    - cannot copy a bridge or tower with 10 blocks: <three years
    - cannot copy a tower of six blocks: <two years
    - cannot copy a tower of three or four blocks: <18 months
    - cannot copy tower of two blocks: <12 months

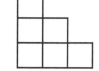

- Speech and language – there may be developmental delay if Thomas:
    - cannot say his birthday or name four colours: <five years
    - cannot say full address, count up to 20: <four years
    - cannot say age, sex, count up to 10: <three years
    - cannot form three-word sentences: <three years
    - cannot follow simple instructions ie. 'Will you get me the ball?': <two years
    - cannot point to named body parts, use simple words like baba, dada etc: <12 months

The second task:

- To assess any single parameter of development:
  - usually speech and language
  - fine motor skills.

This task will need a different approach. You may be told a child's age or alternatively you may be asked to comment on their developmental age.

Quick tip: You should have a well-rehearsed and structured approach to complete the task:

- Always have a few tools ready, such as books, blocks or beads. The child may not be interested in blocks but may engage with books.

- Do not repeatedly try to make a child do things which they are not keen to. You will lose their attention, interest, valuable time and marks.

- Do not keep more than one tool/object in field of vision as multiple objects will distract the child.

- Once you get the child engaged with blocks or books, keep challenging them as far as possible.

- Do not attempt to make the child do all the tasks you have learnt. Your aim here is to arrive at his development age rather than make the child do the entire range of tasks, which is practically never achievable.

The third task:

- To comment on a child's developmental status, for example:
  - he is likely to have global development delay
  - she may be on the autistic spectrum.

Quick tip: A holistic approach is needed here. Normative assessments should be supported by observations. With an autistic child, the examiner will be fully aware that in a five to seven-minute station it is almost impossible to arrive at a diagnosis, but they would like you to pick up some clues such as unusual ways of playing, repetitive body movements, hyperactive behaviour etc.

Details of normative assessments are available in many text books. In the appendix there is a quick reference range for each area that you can use as a skeleton to build on in your preparation.

Practise, practise, practise

To score well in the examination you need to demonstrate an organised approach to developmental assessment – and the best thing you can do to improve your skills is to assess as many children as possible:

- Start with children who are co-operative and do not have any evident developmental delay. Follow a clear and systematic pattern.

- Try to do all of this with the child sitting at a small table.

- Clear all items from the work surface away.

- Bring out one tool/item at a time.

- Remove the item from sight each time before moving on to the next one.

- Demonstrate, where appropriate ie. use a crayon to draw a line and ask the child to copy it.

- Do not leave lots of different items on the table to distract the child, which is a recipe for disaster.

Show the examiners that you have done this before and understand what you would expect of the child. If the child is unable to perform/complete the task set, make things simpler and comment on the gaps in ability.

Within each developmental category it should be possible for you to define developmental age to within two to three months before two years of age and within four to six months between two and five years of age. Interpretation of the developmental assessment should be made with regard to the range of normal findings and in the context of a child's illness or other associated condition.

Trainees who have experience of community paediatrics are at an advantage in terms of developmental assessments, knowledge of support in the community and the various allowances available, but in reality this is not mandatory. You can improve your skills with regular practise with children you come across, and by attending community paediatric sessions. Practise developmental assessment every day with at least one child. The more you interact with children and are able to engage them with blocks, crayons or books to complete set tasks, the more your confidence and familiarity will come across in the exam.

Common sense advice for preparing for the examination is to arrange to attend as many sessions as feasible at your local child development centre (CDC) for an overview. Spend time with multidisciplinary teams, consultants in their clinics, physiotherapists and occupational therapists during various sessions.

Observe, make mental and physical notes and have any doubts clarified. If possible, carry out developmental assessments in their presence and get feedback. Remember, your performance can only get better.

You may be asked by the examiner to assess vision and/or hearing for different age groups. Although these are less likely, you should still be well prepared and your theoretical knowledge should be up to date.

Children with special needs

Children with special needs may have concerns/difficulties with:

- physical impairment – problems with mobility, co-ordination or articulation (dyspraxia)
- sensory impairment – sight/hearing
- speech/language difficulties – delay/articulation/stuttering
- learning disabilities – moderate to severe
- a specific learning disability – dyslexia (reading), writing/numeracy
- emotional difficulties – autism, anxiety, fear, depression
- behavioural difficulties – attention deficit hyperactivity disorder, aggression
- medical condition – asthma, cystic fibrosis, diabetes, chronic renal failure etc.
- global developmental disorder – Down's syndrome, Rett's syndrome, cerebral palsy etc.

CDCs are special, designated areas in children's departments in hospitals or in the community where children with multiple and complex needs are treated. Here, various specialists (doctors, therapists, health visitors and social workers) work together in multidisciplinary teams to provide the necessary care.

They provide specialist help with:

- physiotherapy
- speech and language therapy
- occupational therapy
- home learning scheme ie. portage
- equipment and special aid

- financial support, personal care/mobility etc.
- toy libraries
- specialist play groups, opportunity groups
- respite care
- nurseries, school nurseries, classes.

Using this section

In the following pages you will be presented in the first box with some brief information about a case, and then supplied with a detailed description of an examination, including what you check for and notice in the second box. You are then asked to summarise your findings to the 'examiner', who will be played by a role-player. What is expected of the candidate and ideal findings are then listed in the third box.

If you are working with a study partner, you should read the examination details and discuss your findings with your partner while they have access to these findings and you do not. If you are working alone, either formulate your findings in your head or write them down before checking them against the findings in the third box.

Child development station: case 1

Speech delay – isolated

Information given to the candidate

You are a GP. On entering the station, the examiner introduces you to Anna.

Anna is three years old and she has come to see you with her mother, Joan. She has been referred by her health visitor as the staff at her playgroup are concerned about her speech.

Your task

Assess Anna's speech development.

You have nine minutes; there will be a warning bell at seven minutes.

Examination

You introduce yourself to Anna's mother, obtain her consent to examine her child and inform her that your hands have been thoroughly cleaned. You greet Anna.

You note that Anna is sitting in a corner of the room. She is holding a pencil using her thumb and first two fingers and trying to draw something. She looks apprehensive and moves closer to her mother as you approach her.

You introduce yourself to Anna. She looks shy. You approach the table and ask her name. She does not reply. On your behalf, her mother asks her name. She mumbles something that you cannot understand.

At this stage you can ask Joan to choose a book for Anna that she might be interested in:

- You show the book to Anna and she seems to be interested. You point to different objects in the book and ask her if she knows them. She still does not answer you. You once again seek her mother's help. She responds to her mother and starts naming the objects.

- You note that she has got a good vocabulary. Gradually she responds to you and answers simple questions such as 'Can you show me the cat?' or 'What's the baby is doing?' etc.

- You note she knows the basic colours and she can count 10 objects from the picture book. Slowly, Anna becomes more chatty and carries on a conversation with you.

Diploma in Child Health: Volume 1 © Pavilion Publishing and Media Ltd and its licensors 2014.

- You note that although Anna has a good vocabulary, there is a problem with articulation as she pronounces dog as 'og', door as 'or', and water as 'oter'.
- You ask her mother if she is aware of this. She says that her health visitor has also referred her to a speech specialist for this.
- Looking at the paper you see that she was drawing a man with eyes and lips.

You investigate Anna's gross motor skills further with Joan ie. whether she can ride a tricycle or climb stairs etc:

- She informs you that Anna is toilet trained.
- Anna eats with spoon and fork.
- She drinks from her own cup.

After checking with the examiner you briefly ask her mother about her birth history, any history of tongue tie, significant past medical history or any family history specifically related to speech problems.

During this conversation you note that Anna goes to the corner of the room where she discovers a doll and excitedly calls to her mother and points to it. Joan calls her by name and she runs toward her with the doll and hugs her.

You turn toward the examiner and summarise your findings. You will be notified when there is one minute left.

Findings

- Anna is a lovely three-year-old girl.
- She does not have any dysmorphic features. She does not have a hearing aid.
- She is interested in toys and pictures.
- She responds to her name.
- She can name basic colours.
- She has a good vocabulary.
- Her receptive speech is age appropriate as she understands simple instructions and responds appropriately.
- She has difficulty with her articulation as she is struggling with the pronunciation of certain words.

Although you did not formally assess her other developmental parameters, they seem to be age appropriate as she is toilet trained, she can draw a circle and she can also feed herself. She interacts with her mother very well. She does not have any obvious problem with vision and hearing.

To conclude, Anna has an isolated speech articulation difficulty and you would refer her to speech and language team for formal assessment.

What is expected from the candidate

The candidate should:

- introduce themself to Anna and her mother and request verbal consent to carry out an examination
- make it known that their hands have been thoroughly cleaned before touching the patient
- make personal observations even before forming a rapport
- keep the patient at ease and give simple and easy to understand commands
- build a rapport with the patient
- take advantage of Joan's help when necessary
- choose the correct tool for examination ie. a book or blocks
- check Anna's hearing and level of understanding
- comment on different aspects of speech and language development including receptive, expressive etc.
- identify Anna's articulation abnormality
- assess other parameters briefly before drawing conclusions
- address any concerns Anna's mother might have
- discuss with the examiner other speech problems and their management and refer Anna to the SALT (Speech And Language Therapy) team.

Further information

Parallel play is when toddlers play by themselves, standing or sitting next to another, and is typical of most kids around two years of age. Group play and sharing doesn't usually evolve until age three.

The ability to ride a tricycle and/or bike is an important milestone that most children reach by the time they are about three years old.

By age four, most children can ride a two-wheeled bike with training wheels, which they can take off by the time they are five to six years old.

Most children can count to 10 or more once they are about five and a half years old.

For your notes and thoughts

Child development station: case 2

Fine motor assessment

Information given to the candidate

On entering the station, the examiner introduces you to Asin.

Asin has come with her mother, Sabrina Beckham. Asin is sitting in a wheel chair. She looks to be around six years old.

She is seen by a CDC team regularly.

Your task

Assess Asin's fine motor development.

You are allowed to talk to the patient but are not allowed to ask any history unless allowed by the examiner.

You have nine minutes to complete the station; a warning bell will be given at seven minutes.

The examination

You introduce yourself to Asin's mother and obtain her consent to examine Asin, and inform her that you have thoroughly washed your hands. You greet Asin.

You note that Asin is sitting in a wheelchair comfortably. She has been stabilised by a back strap and back rest. Her wheelchair is not motor operated. She is comfortable and greets you with smile. Her head looks small. She fiddles with her hands in a stereotyped manner. You introduce yourself to Asin. She looks happy. You ask her name. She replies slowly.

At this stage you ask Asin if she likes to draw. She responds by nodding her head. You can tell her vocabulary is limited. You offer her paper and a crayon. You note:

- She holds the pen in an immature grip. You see as she scribbles horizontally and vertically. You ask her if she can draw a circle. She seems to be interested but gives you a vacant smile. You draw a circle and ask her to copy it. She copies it with the same immature pen grip. You draw a square and ask her to copy it. She tries but cannot finish it. You ask her if she can draw a man but she just scribbles.

- You remove the crayon and paper and get some blocks.

Diploma in Child Health: Volume 1 © Pavilion Publishing and Media Ltd and its licensors 2014.

- She was very happy with the blocks and started playing with them. She managed to place nine blocks vertically.
- She could not, however, build a stair with six blocks but after you demonstrate it she is able to.

You investigate Asin's gross motor skills further with her mother ie. whether she can stand and walk with support etc:

- Asin's mother informs you that she is not toilet trained and still in nappies.
- She can eat with spoon and fork.
- She drinks from her own cup but has an ongoing wringing movement.

After checking with the examiner you briefly ask Asin's mother about her birth history, and you come to know that she had a normal birth history and her milestones were normal till she was nine months old, when she gradually started losing her skills and exhibiting signs of delayed development and regression.

You turn toward the examiner and summarise your findings. You will be notified when there is one minute left.

Findings

- Asin is well nourished but her head looks small.
- You would like to measure her weight, height and head circumference and plot these on the appropriate growth chart.
- She is in a wheelchair and needs back support.
- Her fine motor parameters are suggestive of three years, approximately, as she can copy a circle and copy a stair with six blocks and she is having regular wringing type hand movements.
- Her gross motor and personal social milestones look well behind three years and you decide you need to assess them formally.
- She does not have a hearing aid and she is not wearing glasses.

Asin has gross developmental delay including fine motor delay. In view of the history of developmental regression, with repetitive hand movements, small head and being a female child, she might have Rett's syndrome.

OR

You admit to not being able to give a diagnosis and will refer her for further specialist opinion. However, you should be able to identify the delayed milestones.

What is expected from the candidate

The candidate should:

- introduce themself to Asin and her mother and request verbal consent to carry out the examination
- make it known that hands have been thoroughly washed before touching the patient
- make personal observations even before forming a rapport
- keep the patient at ease and give simple and easy to understand commands
- build a rapport with the patient
- take advantage of Asin's mother's help when necessary
- choose the correct tool for examination ie. blocks, beads, paper and crayon
- identify small head, hand movements etc.
- take appropriate birth history, regression etc. from Asin's mother
- demonstrate the ability to assess other parameters briefly, before drawing conclusions
- address any parental concerns
- be able to discuss with the examiner other differentials of milestone regressions
- discuss the input of multidisciplinary teams
- have a knowledge of Disability Living Allowance
- be aware of respite care availability
- look for social service input.

For your notes and thoughts